Power and Risk in Policymaking

Josephine Adekola

Power and Risk in Policymaking

Understanding Public Health Debates

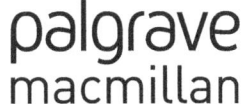

Josephine Adekola
Glasgow Caledonian University
Glasgow, United Kingdom

ISBN 978-3-030-19313-3   ISBN 978-3-030-19314-0 (eBook)
https://doi.org/10.1007/978-3-030-19314-0

© The Editor(s) (if applicable) and The Author(s), under exclusive licence to Springer Nature Switzerland AG 2020
This work is subject to copyright. All rights are solely and exclusively licensed by the Publisher, whether the whole or part of the material is concerned, specifically the rights of translation, reprinting, reuse of illustrations, recitation, broadcasting, reproduction on microfilms or in any other physical way, and transmission or information storage and retrieval, electronic adaptation, computer software, or by similar or dissimilar methodology now known or hereafter developed.
The use of general descriptive names, registered names, trademarks, service marks, etc. in this publication does not imply, even in the absence of a specific statement, that such names are exempt from the relevant protective laws and regulations and therefore free for general use.
The publisher, the authors and the editors are safe to assume that the advice and information in this book are believed to be true and accurate at the date of publication. Neither the publisher nor the authors or the editors give a warranty, express or implied, with respect to the material contained herein or for any errors or omissions that may have been made. The publisher remains neutral with regard to jurisdictional claims in published maps and institutional affiliations.

Cover illustration: Pattern © Melisa Hasan

This Palgrave Pivot imprint is published by the registered company Springer Nature Switzerland AG
The registered company address is: Gewerbestrasse 11, 6330 Cham, Switzerland

Preface

This book looks at the processes of risk communication around public health and safety and considers how policy decisions are made where there is little or no prior scientific understanding of the risk. In particular, the book expands on the understanding of how power and expertise shape risk communication about public health and safety and how policy decisions are shaped as a consequence. The book describes case studies and relied largely upon published sources of data because it was determined that these captured stakeholder inputs, reflected the debates, drew differentially on evidence and experts, would provide greater insight to each of the cases and were more readily comparable across cases. These sources included published peer-reviewed articles, press releases, and government and official reports. The findings suggest that there are several underlying (and salient) mechanisms of power that shape how risk is communicated and, in particular, whose expertise is called upon and whose voices are heard. Further analysis of the cases indicates that 'power' in public health risk communication may be expressed through technical expertise, control of communication and creation of trust (through scientific credibility) such that an argument (within a set of risk arguments) may become amplified (or dominant) in the policy context.

The study contributes to the growing literature on risk communication by advancing knowledge about the role of power and expertise. By analysing the smoking, MMR vaccine and sugar debates through the lens of the policy evaluation risk communication framework (Adekola et al. 2018), this book extends the existing conceptualisation of the social amplification of risk framework from the power and expertise perspective, and to inform the critique of the framework in extant literature.

Glasgow, UK   Josephine Adekola

Reference

Adekola, J, Fischbacher-Smith, D., & Fischbacher-Smith, M. (2018). Light me up: Power and expertise in risk communication and policy-making in the e-cigarette health debates. *Journal of Risk Research.* https://doi.org/10.1080/13669877.2018.1473463. [ABS 2].

Contents

1. Risk, Risk Communication and Policymaking — 1
2. Risk Assessment and the Nature of Expertise in Policy Making — 13
3. A Critique of the Social Amplification of Risk Framework from the Power Perspective — 27
4. The UK Smoking Debate — 43
5. The UK MMR Vaccine Debate — 61
6. The Sugar Debate — 73
7. The Policy Evaluation Risk Communication Framework — 85
8. The Role of Power and Expertise in Social Amplification of Risk — 103
9. Best Practice Risk Communication and Conclusion — 119

Abbreviations

BMJ *British Medical Journal*
CHSC Central Health Services Committee
CMO Chief Medical Officer
EC Electronic cigarette
MH Ministry of Health
MMR Measles, Mumps and Rubella
MRC Medical Research Council
PERC Policy Evaluation Risk Communication
SACCR Standing Advisory Committee on Cancer and Radiotherapy
SARF Social Amplification of Risk Framework
UK United Kingdom
WHO World Health Organization

List of Figures

Fig. 2.1   The process of risk assessment (after Rowe)   16
Fig. 3.1   Policy Evaluation Risk Communication (PERC) framework   37

List of Tables

Table 1.1	Summary of some public health debates in the UK	6
Table 2.1	The different categories of expertise	23
Table 3.1	Elements of social amplification	28
Table 3.2	Dimensions of power in risk communication adapted from the literature	34
Table 7.1	The transition of policy regulation in an evolving risk debate	98
Table 8.1	Hypothetical Scenarios of Social Amplification (or Attenuation) of Risk and Implication for Public Health	114

CHAPTER 1

Risk, Risk Communication and Policymaking

INTRODUCTION

Effective communication is a central part of risk regulation, and it is a key component in helping the public make sense of the risk that they face (Bennett 2010; Fischbacher-Smith et al. 2010; Veland and Aven 2013). It enables people to participate and be heard in decisions about risks that affect them. It is also vital in shaping how policies are formulated and how people understand them and adapt their practices or behaviour as a consequence, to reduce the threat from the risk. Risk communication is the exchange of information about risk (Löfstedt 2008; Veland and Aven 2013) between two or more persons or stakeholder groups, and this may include government agencies, organisations, scientists or individual citizens (Covello et al. 1986). However, risk communication has become the means by which powerful individuals or groups (with vested interest) exploit resources within their means to shape risk arguments and the policy perspective taken thereof (Smith 1988; Warner and Kinslow 2013; Veland and Aven 2013; Demeritt and Nobert 2014; Hardy and Maguire 2016; McKell and De Barro 2016). Yet, the extent to which individuals or public groups use resources within their means to their advantage in risk communication remains an area that has received too little scientific attention.

This book examines the processes of risk communication within the context of the smoking; measles, mumps and rubella (MMR) vaccine; and sugar debates within the UK. It considers how policy decisions are made in times of risk and uncertainty and especially where there is little or no scientific evidence on which to base policy decision-making. Through the lens of the Policy Evaluation Risk Communication (PERC) framework (Adekola et al. 2018), the study analyses the case study of the smoking, MMR vaccine and sugar debates to describe the evolution of risk argument between an initial conceptualisation or identification of the risk to its policy formulation. Within this, the study expands on the role of power and expertise in risk communication, and the evidence from this study has enabled the study to extend the understanding of social amplification of risk from the power perspective.

The understanding of how power and expertise shape risk communication about public health and safety is important because it can reveal underlying yet salient factors that shape public understanding and policy perspectives taken towards risk (which otherwise would go unnoticed or unscrutinised) in ways that may benefit or disadvantage certain public groups. Powerful or resourced stakeholders' groups, for instance, can use the resources within their means to influence the credibility of information flow stations (such as media, technical expertise and educational institutions), which in effect may influence public perception of risk. In addition, they can extend their influence to different response mechanisms of society by introducing bias to individual perception (Lukes 2004) through media such as marketing, advertising, and film and documentary production. There is even the possibility that stakeholder groups may use their influence to engage in relationships with powerful groups, which in turn influences member responses and the type of rationality brought to risk issues (Collingridge and Reeve 1986). Furthermore, powerful groups can also extend their influence to tarnish the reputation of persons or groups who are opposed to their interests by amplifying negative events associated with these people or places in order to reduce their credibility, and therefore any claims made by them.

The analysis carried out in this book is timely, especially in this post-truth[1] era (Keyes 2004; Pazzanese 2016; Flood 2016) where big voices (such as the UK's former justice secretary, Michael Gove or in the case

---

[1] The 'post-truth era' refers to a culture in which facts or evidence are discounted or rendered secondary to emotional appeals; see Keyes, R. 2004. *The post-truth era: Dishonesty and deception in contemporary life*, Macmillan, Pazzanese, C. 2016. Politics in a 'post-truth' age. *Harvard Gazette*, Flood, A. 2016. 'Post-truth' named word of the year by Oxford Dictionaries. *The Guardian*, Tuesday 15 November 2016.

of the United States, Donald Trump) are challenging intellectualism and the role of evidence and experts in making sense of risk issues in times of uncertainty. Gove, in the last days leading up to the UK's EU referendum campaigns, attempted to dissuade the public from expert interpretations (of gloom and doom if Britain exited from the EU) (Brown 2016). He stated that "people in this country have had enough of experts" (Brown 2016). Gove's contention was met with fierce criticism and was immediately challenged, especially by the scientific community. It would, therefore, be interesting to understand the role of experts in shaping our understanding of risk in public health risk communication.

THE CONSTRUCT OF RISK

The term 'risk' is typically associated with unwanted events or outcomes (Renn and Roco 2006) and framed differently by different authors to include an occurrence of an 'adverse event' (Warner et al. 1992), 'loss' (Brearley and Hall 1982) or where 'value is at stake'. The literature identifies three schools of thought: the objective school, the subjective school and one that combines both perspectives. The objective school determines risk by physical facts and believes that what constitutes risk is independent of any bias, assumptions or values (Hansson 2010). However, this assumption has been criticised for ignoring underlying factors (such as personal, structural, institutional and organisational issues) that shape how risk is identified, measured and interpreted (Wynne 1992). The subjective school of thought believes that all risks are socially constructed (Douglas and Wildavsky 1982), and thus an understanding of risk is a reflection of perceived harm or hazard (Slovic and Weber 2002). The core argument here is that our perception of risk cannot be separated from our values, perception and worldview (Gephart et al. 2009). This subjective assumption has, however, been criticised for over-emphasising the 'value' associated with risk (Shrader-Frechette 1991a), and denies that harm does occur whether you believe it or not.

Because of the weaknesses of the first two perspectives of risk, the third perspective combines both objective and subjective elements (Kasperson et al. 1988; Shrader-Frechette 1991b). The assumption made here is that regardless of our subjectivity or the value we place on a risk, risk could pose a real threat or hazard. However, this is only effectively realised when harm is shown to have occurred (Shrader-Frechette 1991a). Shrader-Frechette (1991a) accused the first school of thought of viewing ordinary citizens as ignorant of science and assuming that a technical expert alone has the expertise and ability to make a judgement about the potential risk they face. On the other hand, the subjective school was criticised for assuming that citizens' unwanted behaviour about risk arises because they are a product of biased thinking (Shrader-Frechette 1991a). The strength of the third school of thought is that it recognises the importance of both factual and value components of risk (Shrader-Frechette 1991a) for a robust understanding of risk.

The risk perspective taken in this book aligns with the third school of thought, recognising that while values associated with risk are often issues of perception, the consequences or associated health implications are real. Furthermore, considering that the main aim of this book is to understand how power and expertise shape risk communication processes about public health and safety, the book subscribes to the view that sees risk communication as "a field of play and competition" (Bourdieu 1998) between competing stakeholders' groups (Pidgeon and Barnett 2013; Petts et al. 2001) and where risk arguments are framed in such a way that serves the interest of the stakeholder (Murdock et al. 2003; Pidgeon and Barnett 2013). This definition of risk recognises that risk communication is a process involving both winning an argument and the competition for resources (Adekola et al. 2018).

THE EVOLUTION OF RISK COMMUNICATION

Risk communication has historically been viewed as a process that moves from expert to non-expert, typically referred to as the "deficit model" (Wright and Nerlich 2006; Sturgis and Allum 2004). Irwin and Wynne (2003) termed this model of risk communication the "first order of thinking" that views the public as ignorant; science is presented as speaking the truth to power; scientific claims are often based on the language of certainty; and the diversity and knowledge-ability of the public are ignored by risk managers/communicators. This top-down, one-way model of risk communication has proven to be unsuccessful, as the public has a greater ability to deal with issues of risk than was previously acknowledged (Hansen et al. 2003). Also, one-way model of risk communication has been criticised for failing to open up risk assessment and rationality for public input and scrutiny (Petts 1992). According to Petts et al. (2001), effective risk management requires that control be extended beyond institutional and political control to that of the individual deemed to be at risk. Against this background, there is increasing recognition, and now a general consensus, that risk communication is a two-way, interactive process between communicators and recipients of the message (Shannon 1961; Grönroos 2004).

The "two-way communication model" recognises that feedback is essential in ensuring the effectiveness of the communication (Petts et al. 2001). This, according to Irwin (2014), is a shift to a second order of thinking that encourages greater transparency and public engagement. The transition towards more transparency and engagement has been attributed to the rising recognition and acknowledgement of the benefits of deliberative and participatory democracy and to discussions around the need to invigorate the political and policy processes (Fischer 2003). Irwin (2014) also identified a third order of thinking where there is "more critical reflection–and reflection-informed practice about the relationship between technical change, institutional priorities and wider conceptions of social welfare and justice" (p. 169). Here differences amongst interest groups, including those within scientific communities, are perceived as a resource and less of it been a problem (Stilgoe et al. 2006). This, according to Irwin (2014), "opens up fresh inter-connections between public, scientific, institutional, political and ethical visions of change in all their heterogeneity, conditionality and disagreement" (p. 169). Irwin (2014) remarks that the three different orders of thinking are neither about developing a new toolkit for communication nor about superiority, but rather about examining underlying and fundamental assumptions about how risk is communicated. Ultimately, a choice of first, second or third order of thinking will raise questions around the notion of power and the nature of expertise brought to bear on risk communication in situations of risk and uncertainty.

CONTEXT OF STUDY: PUBLIC DEBATES ABOUT RISK

There has been a significant rise in the number of public debates about risk and safety in recent times. Table 1.1 outlines a few public health debates from the past.

Table 1.1 Summary of some public health debates in the UK

Public health debates	Main issues	References
Smoking	Risk communication about public health and safety around the effects of tobacco. Some argue that smoking is linked to cancer. Those on this side of the argument point to the inadequacies and gaps in the scientific understanding of the risk associated with smoking	Doll and Hill (1950); Van Lancker (1977); Lima and Siegel (1999)
Measles, mumps, rubella	Risk communication about public health and safety around the risk and efficacy of MMR vaccines. A study published in 1998 links the MMR vaccine to rubella, against the dominant view that it was safe for consumption. The study was later dismissed for lack of evidence and faulty interpretation due to an undisclosed interest	Wakefield et al. (1998); Taylor et al. (1999)
Genetically modified food	Risk communication about public health and safety around the use of genetically modified crops in place of conventional ones, and other genetic engineering in food production. Some argue that genetically modified foods can be used to solve the world's food crisis. Others argue that the health implications are not adequately understood, therefore putting public health at risk	Gaskell et al. (1999)
Mobile phones and phone masts	Risk communication about public health and safety around potential health risks of mobile phones and their associated masts. Some claim residents living close to masts complain of health issues ranging from nosebleeds to headaches. Others point to the lack of evidence, as mobile phone use is still in its early stage	Stilgoe (2004); Drake (2010)
Sugar and salt consumption	Risk communication about public health and safety around obesity and other health conditions relating to sugar and salt intake. Some call for government intervention (e.g. higher taxes); others point to the 'nanny state' ideology and the need to leave consumption decisions within individual control	Cordain et al. (2005); He et al. (2008); Grimes et al. (2013)
Electronic cigarettes	Risk communication about public health and safety around the safety and efficacy of electronic cigarettes (EC). Some argue that EC could renormalise smoking, undermining many years of effort de-glamorising smoking. Others argue that EC could save over 50,000 lives a year if people switch from conventional smoking to EC	Cahn and Siegel (2011); Vardavas et al. (2012); McNeill et al. (2015)

Table 1.1 summarises some of the public health communication that has taken place in the UK since 1950. Key features of these emerging debates when they occurred were as follows:

(a) There was a lack of scientific evidence on which to base any rational judgement.
(b) The boundaries and terms of the debates are unclear.
(c) These debates are often characterised by disagreement over fundamental values amongst stakeholder groups.
(d) There are technical disputes about evidence and its interpretation.
(e) There are differences over what precautionary measures to take in mitigating risk, with trade-offs being inevitable.

The rise in public debates about risk has been linked to many factors, and these include the following:

(i) Rapid advancement in ICT that makes access to information and more general interaction possible at almost any time and place.
(ii) Control measures put in place in instances of risk have become a source of risk in themselves (Fischbacher-Smith et al. 2010) because of unforeseen emergent conditions.
(iii) There is also an increasing societal emphasis on corporate social responsibility (CSR) that has shifted the boundaries of CSR in contemporary political life beyond the domain of legality into that of ethics and morality (Irwin 2014), thereby extending the scope of risk debates.

Given the advances in technologies, a more knowledgeable, engaged and aware public, and societal emphasis on CSR, there is the expectation that risk communication (or debates) about public health and safety will continue to be the means of forging public health policymaking, and it is on this basis that this book adopts public health risk debates (communication) as the situational context in which the role of power and expertise in risk communication about public health and safety is investigated.

Structure of Book

This book is structured into nine chapters. Chapter 2 situates the discussion on risk and risk communication within the context of policymaking. It considers the role of expertise in policymaking and emerging debates around technical expertise in policymaking that may amplify or reduce certain perspectives of risk. Chapter 3 provides an account of the social amplification of risk framework (SARF) and then explores key concepts within the literature that can inform a critique of this framework. Chapters 4, 5 and 6 represent the results and analysis chapters of this book and aim empirically to explain how power and expertise shape risk communication and the policy perspective taken on risk. Chapter 7 discusses the findings of the study through the lens of the PERC framework (see Adekola et al. 2018). The implications of the findings for risk communication are also discussed here. Insights from the study enabled the development of the SARF from the power and expertise perspective in Chap. 8. The final chapter (Chap. 9) summarises the study and sets out best practice risk communication for policymakers and the wider stakeholders in the risk arena.

REFERENCES

Adekola, J., Fischbacher-Smith, D., & Fischbacher-Smith, M. (2018). Light me up: Power and expertise in risk communication and policy-making in the e-cigarette health debates. *Journal of Risk Research*, 1–15.

Bennett, P. (2010). *Risk communication and public health*. Oxford: Oxford University Press.

Bourdieu, P. (1998). *Bourdieu: On television and journalism*. London: Pluto Press.

Brearley, C. P., & Hall, M. R. P. (1982). *Risk and ageing*. London: Routledge & Kegan Paul.

Brown, T. (2016). Evidence, expertise, and facts in a "post-truth" society. *British Medical Journal 2016*, 355. https://doi.org/10.1136/bmj.i6467

Cahn, Z., & Siegel, M. (2011). Electronic cigarettes as a harm reduction strategy for tobacco control: A step forward or a repeat of past mistakes & quest. *Journal of Public Health Policy, 32*, 16–31.

Collingridge, D., & Reeve, C. (1986). *Science speaks to power: The role of experts in policy making*. New York: St Martin's press.

Cordain, L., Eaton, S. B., Sebastian, A., Mann, N., Lindeberg, S., Watkins, B. A., O'Keefe, J. H., & Brand-Miller, J. (2005). Origins and evolution of the Western diet: Health implications for the 21st century. *The American Journal of Clinical Nutrition, 81*, 341–354.

Covello, V. T., Slovic, P., & von Winterfeldt, D. (1986). *Risk communication: A review of the literature*. Washington, DC: National Emergency Training Center.

Demeritt, D., & Nobert, S. (2014). Models of best practice in flood risk communication and management. *Environmental Hazards, 13*, 313–328.

Doll, R., & Hill, B. (1950). Smoking and carcinoma of the lung. *British Medical Journal, 2*, 739–748.
Douglas, M., & Wildavsky, A. (1982). How can we know the risks we face? Why risk selection is a social process. *Risk Analysis, 2*, 49–58.
Drake, F. (2010). Protesting mobile phone masts: Risk, neoliberalism, and governmentality. *Science, Technology & Human Values, 36*, 522–548.
Fischbacher-Smith, D., Irwin, A., & Fischbacher-Smith, M. (2010). Bringing light to the shadows and shadows to the light: Risk, risk management, and risk communication. In P. Bennet, K. Calman, S. Curtis, & D. Fischbacher-Smith (Eds.), *Risk communication and public health* (pp. 23–38). Oxford University Press: Oxford. https://doi.org/10.1093/acprof:oso/9780199562848.003.02. ISBN 9780199562848.
Fischer, F. (2003). *Reframing public policy: Discursive politics and deliberative practices*. Oxford: Oxford University Press.
Gaskell, G., Bauer, M. W., Durant, J., & Allum, N. C. (1999). Worlds apart? The reception of genetically modified foods in Europe and the US. *Science, 285*, 384–387.
Gephart, R. P., Van Maanen, J., & Oberlechner, T. (2009). Organizations and risk in late modernity. *Organization Studies, 30*, 141–155.
Grimes, C. A., Riddell, L. J., Campbell, K. J., & Nowson, C. A. (2013). Dietary salt intake, sugar-sweetened beverage consumption, and obesity risk. *Pediatrics, 131*, 14–21.
Grönroos, C. (2004). The relationship marketing process: Communication, interaction, dialogue, value. *Journal of business & Industrial Marketing, 19*(2), 99–113.
Hansen, J., Holm, L., Frewer, L., Robinson, P., & Sandøe, P. (2003). Beyond the knowledge deficit: Recent research into lay and expert attitudes to food risks. *Appetite, 41*(2), 111–121. https://doi.org/10.1016/S0195-6663(03)00079-5
Hansson, S. O. (2010). Risk: Objective or subjective, facts or values. *Journal of Risk Research, 13*, 231–238.
Hardy, C., & Maguire, S. (2016). Organizing risk: Discourse, power, and "riskification". *Academy of Management Review, 41*, 80–108.
He, F. J., Marrero, N. M., & MacGregor, G. A. (2008). Salt intake is related to soft drink consumption in children and adolescents a link to obesity? *Hypertension, 51*, 629–634.
Irwin, A. (2014). From deficit to democracy (re-visited). *Public Understanding of Science, 23*, 71–76.
Irwin, A., & Wynne, B. (Eds.). (2003). *Misunderstanding science?: The public reconstruction of science and technology*. Cambridge: Cambridge University Press.
Kasperson, R. E., Renn, O., Slovic, P., Brown, H. S., Emel, J., Goble, R., Kasperson, J. X., & Ratick, S. (1988). The social amplification of risk: A conceptual framework. *Risk Analysis, 8*, 177–187.

Lima, J. C., & Siegel, M. (1999). The tobacco settlement: An analysis of newspaper coverage of a national policy debate, 1997–98. *Tobacco Control, 8*, 247–253.
Löfstedt, R. (2008). *Risk management in post-trust societies*. London: Earthscan.
Lukes, S. (2004). *Power: A radical view*. London: Macmillan International Higher Education.
McKell, S., & De Barro, P. (2016). Between two absolutes lies risk: Risk communication in biosecurity discourse. In *Communicating Risk* (pp. 229–241). London: Palgrave Macmillan.
McNeill, A., Brose, L. S., Calder, R., Hitchman, S. C., Hajek, P., & McRobbie, H. (2015). E-cigarettes: An evidence update. A report commissioned by Public Health England. *Public Health England*. www.gov.uk/government/uploads/system/uploads/attachment_data/file/454516/Ecigarettes_an_evidence_update_A_report_commissioned_by_Public_Health_England.pdf. Accessed 22 Aug 2015.
Murdock, G., Petts, J., & Horlick-Jones, T. (2003). After amplification: Rethinking the role of the media in risk communication. In *The social amplification of risk* (pp. 156–178). London: Earthscan.
Petts, J. (1992). Incineration risk perceptions and public concern: Experience in the UK improving risk communication. *Waste Management & Research, 10*(2), 169–182.
Petts, J., Horlick-Jones, T., Murdock, G., Hargreaves, D., McLachlan, S., & Lofstedt, R. (2001). *Social amplification of risk: The media and the public*. Sudbury: HSE Books.
Pidgeon, N., & Barnett, J. (2013). *Chalara and the social amplification of risk*. London: Department for Environment, Food and Rural Affairs.
Renn, O., & Roco, M. C. (2006). Nanotechnology and the need for risk governance. *Journal of Nanoparticle Research, 8*, 153–191.
Shannon, C. E. (1961). Two-way communication channels. In *Proceedings of the Fourth Berkeley Symposium on Mathematical Statistics and Probability, Volume 1: Contributions to the Theory of Statistics*. Oakland: The Regents of the University of California.
Shrader-Frechette, K. (1991a). *Reductionist approaches to risk*. New York: Oxford University Press.
Shrader-Frechette, K. S. (1991b). *Risk and rationality: Philosophical foundations for populist reforms*. Oxford: University of California Press.
Slovic, P., & Weber, E. U. (2002). *Perception of risk posed by extreme events*. Center for Decision Sciences (CDS) working paper Columbia University 2002.
Smith, D. (1988). *Corporate power, risk assessment and the control of major hazards: A study of Canvey Island and Ellesmere Port*. Manchester: University of Manchester.
Stilgoe, J. (2004). *Experts and anecdotes: Shaping the public science of mobile phone health risks*. PhD dissertation, University College London.

Stilgoe, J., Irwin, A., & Jones, K. (2006). *The received wisdom: Opening up expert advice.* London: Demos.

Sturgis, P., & Allum, N. (2004). Science in society: Re-evaluating the deficit model of public attitudes. *Public Understanding of Science, 13*(1), 55–74. https://doi.org/10.1177/0963662504042690

Taylor, B., Miller, E., Farrington, C., Petropoulos, M. C., Favot-Mayaud, I., Li, J., & Waight, P. A. (1999). Autism and measles, mumps, and rubella vaccine: No epidemiological evidence for a causal association. *The Lancet, 353*(9169), 2026–2029.

Van Lancker, J. L. (1977). Smoking and disease. *NIDA Research Monograph, 17*, 230–288.

Vardavas, C. I., Anagnostopoulos, N., Kougias, M., Evangelopoulou, V., Connolly, G. N., & Behrakis, P. K. (2012). Short-term pulmonary effects of using an electronic cigarette: Impact on respiratory flow resistance, impedance, and exhaled nitric oxide. *Chest Journal, 141*, 1400–1406.

Veland, H., & Aven, T. (2013). Risk communication in the light of different risk perspectives. *Reliability Engineering & System Safety, 110*, 34–40.

Wakefield, A. J., Murch, S. H., Anthony, A., Linnell, J., Casson, D. M., Malik, M., Berelowitz, M., Dhillon, A. P., Thomson, M. A., Harvey, P., & Valentine, A. (1998). RETRACTED: Ileal-lymphoid-nodular hyperplasia, non-specific colitis, and pervasive developmental disorder in children. *Lancet, 351*(9103), 637–641.

Warner, K. D., & Kinslow, F. (2013). Manipulating risk communication: Value predispositions shape public understandings of invasive species science in Hawaii. *Public Understanding of Science, 22*, 203–218.

Warner, V., Weissman, M., Fendrich, M., Wickramaratne, P., & Moreau, D. (1992). The course of major depression in the offspring of depressed parents: Incidence, recurrence, and recovery. *Archives of General Psychiatry, 49*, 795–801.

Wright, N., & Nerlich, B. (2006). Use of the deficit model in a shared culture of argumentation: The case of foot and mouth science. *Public Understanding of Science, 15*(3), 331–342. https://doi.org/10.1177/0963662506063017

Wynne, B. (1992). Carving out science (and politics) in the regulatory jungle. *Social Studies of Science, 22*(4), 745–758. https://doi.org/10.1177/030631292022004011

CHAPTER 2

Risk Assessment and the Nature of Expertise in Policy Making

PUBLIC HEALTH POLICYMAKING

Public health policy has significant implications for human health in general (Brownson et al. 2009) and defines the ways in which public health issues are framed, viewed and accepted in the political agenda, a process rooted within risk communication. Dewey (1927) defines public policy as the public and its problem and Dye (1992) views this simply as what government chooses to do or not to do. A broader definition is that of Peters (2015), who conceptualises public policy as the sum of government activities carried out directly or indirectly, and which affect or have consequences for the daily life of people within society. Thomas and Grindle (1990), for instance, describe a simple and linear approach to policy development in which policy development starts from setting the policy agenda, and then moves to decision and implementation. The alternative approach is the non-linear approach to policy development that requires that (a) risk is framed within the wider international, national and local contexts (Holland et al. 2004) and (b) input from different public groups is considered in such a way that reflects modern-day evolutionary and interactive policymaking, especially when confronted with issues of ambiguity, complexity and uncertainty. However, regardless of which approach is adopted, public health issues are rife with complexity and ambiguity.

© The Author(s) 2020
J. Adekola, *Power and Risk in Policymaking*,
https://doi.org/10.1007/978-3-030-19314-0_2

The Nature of the Problem in Public Health Risk

Public health risk, like many other forms of risk, is confronted with issues of ambiguity, complexity and uncertainty (Renn et al. 2011), and these are the key concepts underlying the transition of risk argument in a policy debate.

Ambiguity

Ambiguity is a situation where there are multiple legitimate viewpoints about risk. This may be a result of different justification, or the broader meanings attributed to a perceived threat or risk (Stirling 2003). This means that there are two types of ambiguity—interpretive and normative (Renn and Klinke 2015). Interpretive ambiguity arises from differences in legitimate interpretation. This typically occurs when issues are viewed through different lenses. For example, the interpretation of an issue when it is viewed from an economic perspective is different from when viewed from the public health or moral perspective. Normative ambiguity arises from disagreement about priorities, assumptions and values (Renn and Klinke 2015). The problem that ambiguity creates in a risk communication is the multiple legitimate interpretations that are brought to bear on the risk issue compounded by multiple vested interests competing to legitimise their own argument among others. Thus, this further politicises the decision-making process and any resultant policy formulation.

Complexity

The issue of complexity is exemplified by emergent conditions associated with risk. Complexity is defined as the difficulty in understanding the causal relationship between multiple factors and adverse effects (Underdal 2010). This difficulty may arise from tight coupling of the system (Perrow 2011), an interaction of a set of complex multi-causal factors (Klinke and Renn 2002), the length of time between cause and effect, local variation, and other external intervening variables (Renn et al. 2011). A non-linear relationship may also be experienced where cause and effect relationships do not follow a linear pattern, due to the emergent nature of the risk, or errors in the understanding of the risk that are typical of emergent forms of risk and diseases (Fischbacher-Smith and Calman 2010).

Uncertainty

Uncertainty arises as a result of limited or a complete lack of scientific knowledge that creates problems around risk calculative practices, especially in determining the likelihood of a risk occurring and the consequences thereof (Renn 2008; Filar and Haurie 2010). Renn (2008) distinguishes uncertainty based on five components: (1) *variability*—different target of existing vulnerabilities; (2) *inferential effect*—modelling errors; (3) *indeterminacy*—different interpretation in the cause and effect relationship due to variation in a random event; (4) *systematic boundaries*—focusing on a limited parameter; and (5) *ignorance*—lack or absence of knowledge. Renn and Klinke (2015) explain that while the first two components are epistemological issues that can be resolved with improved knowledge and better re-modelling techniques, the last three components are genuinely uncertain and can only be characterised with a scientific approach but not necessarily resolved by it.

The nature of problems in public health risk, as identified above, suggests that risk communication is embedded within a larger societal context complicated by ambiguity, complexity and uncertainty. This creates a conducive environment for resources to be exploited by powerful groups, with a bid to dominate the risk communication arena. The less disadvantaged groups are often left to bear the consequences of any misunderstanding in the perspective taken on the risk.

RISK ASSESSMENT

Risk assessment is generally seen as the probability of an unwanted event occurring (Renn and Sellke 2011), which means that risk assessment involves the use of prior evidence to make a valuable judgement about risk. Risk assessment is defined as "the process of estimating and evaluating risk, understood as the possibility of beneficial and harmful outcomes and the likelihood of their occurrence in a stated timescale" (Titterton 2004, p. 83). It is also defined as the "probability distribution or similar quantification that describes uncertainty about the magnitudes, timing or nature of possible health and environmental consequences associated with possible exposure to specified substance, processes, actions or events" (Covello and Merkhoher 2013, p. 3).

This means that risk assessment involves both technical analysis and social evaluation of the nature, magnitude and likelihood of a risk occurring

(Slovic 1999). The technical evaluation is typically a scientific process carried out by technical expertise and often tends to have more significance than the social evaluation of the risk, especially in the policy domain (Jasanoff 2009). This traditional model of risk assessment (where there is large reliance on technical experts) is seen as effective where the information is complete and where there is prior evidence. However, in situations involving a new or emerging risk arena, the processes of risk assessment become disputable as there is little prior evidence to carry out effective technical risk analysis. The limitation of the traditional model of risk assessment, especially in a new and emerging form of risk, led to a suggested model (Fig. 2.1), adapted by both Irwin et al. (1982) and Fischbacher-Smith et al. (2010), which goes back to the work of Rowe (1977) on "anatomy of risk".

The process of risk assessment model after Rowe (1977), adapted by both Irwin et al. (1982) and Fischbacher-Smith et al. (2010), separates the processes around risk analysis (technical process) from risk acceptability (social process). The core value of this model is that it recognises the input of both technical and local expertise, especially where there is a weak evidential base to make valuable technical judgements. This socio-technical process recognises that those potentially at risk or in close proximity to various hazardous locations may have valuable insight into the nature of the risk, and this could be useful in bridging the knowledge gap or in providing new information about risk.

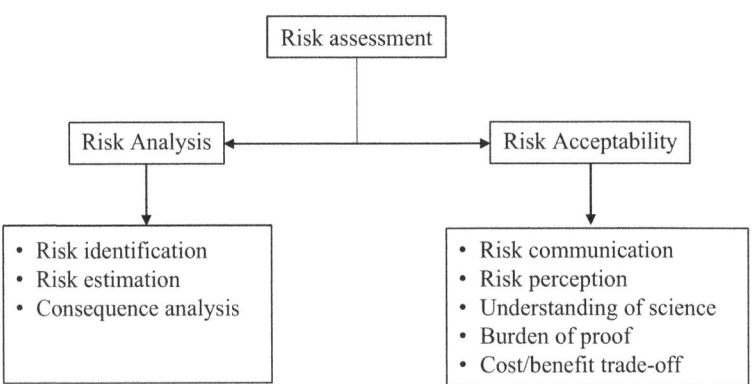

Fig. 2.1 The process of risk assessment (after Rowe). (Source: Fischbacher-Smith et al. 2010, p. 28)

This adapted model avoids the "pitfalls of individualism" and enhances the ability of policymakers and risk regulators to deal with "wicked problems" (Rittel and Webber 1973) while enhancing its risk acceptability. Wicked problems are issues that are difficult to resolve because they are difficult to clearly define and are associated with unforeseen consequences that are politically and socially complex (trans-scientific issues) (Grint 2010). Where 'wicked' problems exist, as they do in many public health risk issues, the use of such an interactive and collaborative (Weber and Khademian 2008) socio-technical approach would produce a more effective solution to complex policy problems that require complex solutions.

Practical Logic of Policy Evaluation Framework

Fischer (2003), in an attempt to advance knowledge of a socio-technical policy approach, developed a practical logic of the policy evaluation framework. The framework looks at how knowledge is incorporated into policy processes and describes how a set of policy arguments transitions between technical evaluation and normative evaluation. The framework identifies four levels in this transition (Fischer 1995, p. 243): the technical analytical discourse (technical verification), situational validation, societal vindication and ideological choice. These four layers are set in such a way that the process of technical verification is influenced by and influences those normative processes of local validation and societal vindication that determine the outcomes of ideological choices made by policymakers (Fischbacher-Smith 2012).

Technical evaluation of the risk is carried out at the technical verification stage to clarify on what is known, and on areas of uncertainty (Fischer 2003). Disagreement may exist between different expert and public groups based on available evidence and its interpretation, as the debate here determines where the burden of proof lies (Fischbacher-Smith 2012). The outcome of the technical verification then leads to evaluation and social construction that raises questions of validation and whether a particular line of argument can be adopted in a local context; "validation is an interpretive process of reasoning that takes place within the framework of the normative belief systems brought to bear on the problem situation" (p. 21) and discussed within the societal context where the problem lies. Processes around situational validation and societal vindication then shape the ideological choice made by policymakers (Fischer 2003). Fischbacher-Smith (2012) explain that technical analysis of risk takes place between the processes of technical verification and situational validation. The risk acceptability debate takes place between the processes of situational validation and social vindication, and, as we move towards social vindication and ideological choice, the risk debate becomes more politicised, and political power is perceived more as shaping the risk arguments (Fischbacher-Smith 2012).

The practical logic of policy evaluation framework is useful in terms of shedding light on how technical and normative discourse interacts in deliberative and socio-technical policymaking. However, the framework did not explain the outcome of science and expertise in policymaking. It is in this arena that Collingridge and Reeve's (1986) under-critical and over-critical models become useful. The under-critical and over-critical models more explicitly set out the outcome of the science—policy relationship that describes how scientific experts influence policymaking.

Under-Critical Model and Over-Critical Model

The over-critical and under-critical models assume that there is an unhappy marriage between science and policymaking. The core argument is that science has a very marginal influence on policy decisions and is often used to back up or refute arguments on policy perspectives that have already been decided (Collingridge and Reeve 1986). In the under-critical model, scientific evidence is received with little or no open criticism because (a) powerful interests determine what is legitimate science and what is not; (b) little or no scrutiny is given to scientific facts that fit with existing policy, ideology and interests; (c) the argument is already institutionalised in policy practices, even though it might be uncertain; and (d) there may be suppression of other scientific conjectures which threaten policy consensus (Collingridge and Reeve 1986). In this scenario, there is greater influence of political power shaping how science and expertise is received and accepted (Fischbacher-Smith 2012).

The over-critical model is where disagreements exist within the scientific community and where those with power cannot suppress or constrain other perspectives because (a) the evidence base is weak or inconclusive; (b) scientific evidence presented by different groups of experts is subjected to intense scrutiny with the aim of undermining the evidence of the other; and (c) there are challenges associated with interdisciplinary risk problems, which lead to different and conflicting worldviews. In the over-critical model, less political power is perceived to determine the outcome of technical evidence (Fischbacher-Smith 2012). The result is an endless technical debate, which could carry on as long as actors involved are motivated and interested in remaining in the debate. The over-critical and under-critical models described by Collingridge and Reeve (1986) provide useful insight into how technical expertise is incorporated into policymaking. The nature of political power within this is made explicit by Fischbacher-Smith (2012). However, what Collingridge and Reeve (1986) did not do was shed light on how, in an evolving policy debate, arguments transition from one model to the other (Fischbacher-Smith 2012).

Fischbacher-Smith (2012) argues that the over-critical and under-critical models are two ends of a continuum that leave the understanding of the negotiation of policy arguments between them unclear and poorly documented. The negotiation of policy arguments between the under-critical and overcritical models is an essential *gap* in the literature that needs to be filled. This is the context of this book. This will help advance understanding of how a certain policy perspective becomes dominant and legitimised in a policy context, especially where multi-interpretation, values and strong power dynamics are brought to bear in policy debates relating to risk. Policy inquiry relating to risk is a process at the forefront of science and technical expertise in shaping public understanding and policy perspectives taken on the risk. Therefore, understanding the construct of 'expertise' and emerging debates within this literature becomes essential, especially when dealing with interdisciplinary public health risk issues that are further associated with uncertainty, ambiguity and complexity.

Expertise

Technical experts are key influential agents in helping the public make sense of the risk that they face (Fischbacher-Smith 2012), both in the technical analysis of the risk and in the interpretation of its meaning within a social context (social evaluation of risk). They are important for two main reasons. First, scientific expertise is often perceived as a credible source and is therefore more likely to be believed. However, this does not always translate into public uptake of scientific advice, as "known sources" are also powerful sources that impact upon public uptake of risk information (Adekola et al. 2017). Second, technical experts help the public process risk information through various communication outlets, as they often have the requisite knowledge to decode the meaning in scientific information. While this is advantageous in terms of aiding end users in making sense of the risk information, the negative implication of this is that where there are vested interests or reputational issues, risk information may be subjected to distortion, amplifying or reducing certain aspects of the risk. Hence, this may impact on how risk messages are decoded, transmitted and received. As a result, technical experts are key influential actors in shaping the understanding of risk since they play central roles in identifying, negotiating and communicating risk.

Traditionally, the definition of experts in the literature tends to favour a scientifically recognised expertise over other types of expertise which are typically classed as 'lay knowledge'. For example, an expert is defined as a person who "no longer relies on an analytical principle (rule, guideline, and maxim) to connect understanding of a situation to an appropriate action" (Benner 1984, p. 127) and who focuses on connecting underlying ideologies and principles to make meaning (Cross 2004). For Neils Bohr, an expert is a person who has made all the mistakes there are to make in a very small field (cited in Otway 1987). The issue of contention within the arena of expertise lies in how technical expertise is seen as superior to other forms of knowledge, and also in whose scientific evidence is interpreted and communicated.

Evidence and Scientific Interpretation of the Risk

Within the literature, a number of important issues have been raised that may influence how evidence or risk signals are interpreted by experts, such that a certain perception of risk may become amplified or reduced. These are discussed below.

- *Conflicting and longstanding disciplinary practices:* Many public health risks are interdisciplinary risk issues. Thus, there are often conflicts in longstanding disciplinary practices and norms, such as epistemological and ontological differences that affect the nature of the scientific disputes that arise in risk communication.
- *Domain specificity:* These is the increasing recognition that expertise is domain specific (Schneider et al. 1989; McGraw and Pinney 1990; Smith and McCloskey 2000; Castel et al. 2007), and as such, the reliability of such expertise diminishes as we move outside of that domain (Fischbacher-Smith 2012). This is because the exercise of technical expertise outside the appropriate domain may lead to error

in the understanding of the nature of the risk due to, for example, 'intrusions' (Castel et al. 2007). Intrusion is interpreting domain-related information that may be unrelated to the risk concerned (Castel et al. 2007) and this may amplify (or attenuate) certain aspects of the risk with domain-related information. The implication of this is that it may lead to inadequacies or errors in the understanding of the nature of risk that could be problematic for risk managers in managing the risk and its emergent properties.
- *Paradigm blindness:* The issue of paradigm blindness is also raised in the literature and this describes a situation where experts are either unable or unwilling to accept alternative worldviews (Edelsky 1990; Fischbacher-Smith 2012). Collingridge and Reeve (1986) have suggested that an expert's worldview is often left unchanged as long as evidence exists to support it. The challenge here, however, is where evidence becomes politicised and in a way that prevents an expert (who is an important sense-making aid in risk communication) from seeing (or attenuating the significance of) other alternative worldviews beyond their own.
- *Vested interest and bias:* Vested interests may impact on expert judgement and interpretation (Fischbacher-Smith 2012) and lead to motivational bias (Tversky and Kahneman 1974; Slovic 1999; Shrader-Frechette 1996). Vested interests often times do expose an expert to powerful interest groups that may use them to their own advantage, especially as many public health risk debates occur in situations of uncertainty.
- *Institutional, structural and organisational culture or conditions:* There is also a debate about how experts are trained and developed that has implications for how evidence is interpreted (Fischbacher-Smith 2012). Fischbacher-Smith (2012), for instance, argue that expertise is shaped by a set of overlapping networks of structures (e.g. professional, organisational, national and international dimensions) and these impact on how experts are trained, validated and developed over time in such a way that shapes their behaviour, worldview and the attitude they take to risk. Where there is vested interest, institutional or organisational rules and principles may be intentionally positioned to produce certain effects in the worldview, attitude and behaviour of experts, and hence the interpretation they bring to bear on risk (Fischbacher-Smith 2012).

The issues discussed here raise important issues around the extent to which we can trust and rely on technical expertise in policy debate about risk, especially where there is a weak evidential base. More importantly, it calls for accountability of technical expertise in risk communication about public health and safety, especially where the science is contested. It is at this juncture that other expertise such as local expertise (or experiences) may play a significant role in enhancing the accountability of technical expertise in risk communication.

The Alternative View: Categorising Expertise

The alternative option in situations of risk and uncertainty is to view technical expertise as one form of expertise in the midst of many in risk communication and policy inquiry relating to risk, rather than one taken as absolute in the judgement of risk that shapes the policy perspective taken on it. Moreover, there is the so-called citizen's science argument (Irwin 2015) where experiential knowledge and expertise is seen as equally valuable in shaping the understanding of risk, especially where there are gaps in scientific knowledge. This is in no way aimed to undermine the significance of technical expertise in risk communication about public health and safety, but rather to emphasise that the public health risk policy arena is by no means reliant on any singular form of expertise. The core argument here is that there is a place for technical expertise and also other forms of expertise (such as experiential expertise) in risk communication about public health and safety. Technical expertise can be relied upon when confronted by 'knowns' (although there are 'unknown unknowns'), and in static and predictable situations (assuming the stakes are not high). This is not necessarily the case in an emerging risk scenario, where the knowledge about a risk and its emergence is largely unknown. In a new and emerging risk arena, there is a greater need for a socio-technical approach to risk assessment and policymaking where the input of all stakeholders (including ordinary citizens) is equally valued and weighted in policy decision-making.

The Different Categories of Expertise

Hoppe (2010) makes a distinction between a technical expert and a public expert (technocrat) that forms the first two categories of expertise. According to Hoppe (2010), a 'technical expert' is an expert recognised as a qualified scientist who works within the rigour of scientific methodology

Table 2.1 The different categories of expertise

Technical experts (Ziman 2002)	Public expert/ technocrat (Hoppe 2010)	Industry/corporate experts (Collingridge and Reeve 1986)	Local/experiential expertise (Alan Irwin 2002)
Authoritative or recognised scientists who work in knowledge institutions	Scientists who work in public offices (e.g. Chief Scientific Officer)	Scientists who work for corporations (e.g. a chemist working for a pharmaceutical company)	Ordinary citizens who are experts in their daily routine (e.g. local farmers, mothers)

in a specific field and who has received specialised training in an institution of higher education (Suleiman 1977). A 'public expert' (or technocrat), on the other hand, is a technical expert who works in public offices or government institutions (e.g. Chief Scientific Officer) and whose role is to support government in achieving its aims and objectives. The third category of expertise is that of 'industry experts'. This group comprises technical experts who work for corporations or industry (e.g. a chemist working for the tobacco industry), and whose interest is in protecting the interest of the corporation or industry for which they work. The final category of expertise is termed 'citizen's scientist' (Irwin 2002) or experiential expertise. This form of expertise is based on the daily life experiences of individuals or groups. This may include local farmers, mothers or those in close proximity to a risk location or hazard (see Table 2.1).

Having distinguished these four categories, it must be noted that there is the possibility that one person may fit into all these four categories. Spruijt et al. (2014) suggested that the role of experts is influenced by context, type of problem and personal values. This means that the platform in which a type of expertise is expressed (as technical, public or industry or local expertise) may determine the nature of interpretation brought to bear on risk signal or evidence. It is therefore important to declare affiliation when interpreting risk signals, and this should be taken into consideration during associated policymaking.

References

Adekola, J., Fischbacher-Smith, M., Fischbacher-Smith, D., & Adekola, O. (2017). Health risks from environmental degradation in the Niger Delta, Nigeria. *Environment and Planning C: Politics and Space, 35*, 334–354.

Benner, P. (1984). From novice to expert. *American Journal of Nursing, 82*(3), 402–407.

Brownson, R. C., Chriqui, J. F., & Stamatakis, K. A. (2009). Understanding evidence-based public health policy. *American Journal of Public Health, 99,* 1576–1583.

Castel, A. D., McCabe, D. P., Roediger, H. L., & Heitman, J. L. (2007). The dark side of expertise domain-specific memory errors. *Psychological Science, 18,* 3–5.

Collingridge, D., & Reeve, C. (1986). *Science speaks to power: The role of experts in policy making.* London: Pinter.

Covello, V. T., & Merkhoher, M. W. (2013). *Risk assessment methods: Approaches for assessing health and environmental risks.* Berlin: Springer Science & Business Media.

Cross, N. (2004). Expertise in design: An overview. *Design Studies, 25,* 427–441.

Dewey, J. (1927). Search for the great community. In L. A. Hickman & T. M. Alexander (Eds.), *The essential Dewey* (p. 293). Bloomington: Indiana University Press.

Dye, T. R. (1992). *Understanding public policy.* Boston: Pearson.

Edelsky, C. (1990). Whose agenda is this anyway? A response to McKenna, Robinson, and Miller. *Educational Researcher, 19,* 7–11.

Filar, J. A., & Haurie, A. (2010). *Uncertainty and environmental decision making.* New York: Springer.

Fischbacher-Smith, D. (2012). Getting pandas to breed: Paradigm blindness and the policy space for risk prevention, mitigation and management. *Risk Management, 14*(3), 177–201.

Fischbacher-Smith, D., & Calman, K. (2010). A precautionary tale–the role of the precautionary principle in policy making for public health. In *Risk communication and public health* (p. 197). Oxford: Oxford University Press.

Fischbacher-Smith, D., Irwin, A., & Fischbacher-Smith, M. (2010). Bringing light to the shadows and shadows to the light: Risk, risk management, and risk communication. In P. Bennet, K. Calman, S. Curtis, & D. Fischbacher-Smith (Eds.), *Risk Communication and Public Health* (pp. 23–38). Oxford University Press: Oxford. https://doi.org/10.1093/acprof:oso/9780199562848.003.02. ISBN 9780199562848.

Fischer, F. (1995). *Evaluating public policy.* Chicago: Nelson Hall.

Fischer, F. (2003). *Reframing public policy: Discursive politics and deliberative practices.* Oxford: Oxford University Press.

Grint, K. (2010). Wicked problems and clumsy solutions: The role of leadership. In *The new public leadership challenge* (pp. 169–186). London: Palgrave Macmillan.

Holland, W. W., Mossialos, E., Allin, S., McKee, M., & World Health, O. (2004). *Making decisions on public health: A review of eight countries.* Copenhagen: World Health Organization.

Hoppe, R. (2010). From "knowledge use" towards "boundary work": Sketch of an emerging new agenda for inquiry into science-policy interaction. In *Knowledge Democracy* (pp. 169–186). Berlin/Heidelberg: Springer.

Irwin, A. (2002). *Citizen science: A study of people expertise and sustainable development.* London: Routledge.
Irwin, A. (2015). Citizen science and scientific citizenship. In *Science communication today.* Nancy Université.
Irwin, A., Smith, D., & Griffiths, R. (1982). Risk analysis and public policy for major hazards. *Physics in Technology, 13,* 258.
Jasanoff, S. (2009). *The fifth branch: Science advisers as policymakers.* Cambridge, MA: Harvard University Press.
Klinke, A., & Renn, O. (2002). A new approach to risk evaluation and management: Risk-based, precaution-based, and discourse-based strategies. *Risk Analysis, 22,* 1071–1094.
McGraw, K. M., & Pinney, N. (1990). The effects of general and domain-specific expertise on political memory and judgment. *Social Cognition, 8,* 9.
Otway, H. (1987). Experts, risk communication, and democracy. *Risk Analysis, 7,* 125–129.
Perrow, C. (2011). *Normal accidents: Living with high risk technologies.* Princeton: Princeton University Press.
Peters, B. G. (2015). *American public policy: Promise and performance.* Los Angeles: CQ Press.
Petts, J., Horlick-Jones, T., Murdock, G., Hargreaves, D., McLachlan, S., & Lofstedt, R. (2001). *Social amplification of risk: The media and the public.* Sudbury: HSE Books.
Pidgeon, N., & Barnett, J. (2013). *Chalara and the social amplification of risk.* London: Department for Environment, Food and Rural Affairs.
Renn, O. (2008). *Risk governance: Coping with uncertainty in a complex world.* London: Earthscan.
Renn O., & Klinke A. (2015). Risk governance and resilience: New approaches to cope with uncertainty and ambiguity. In U. Fra. Paleo. (Eds.), *Risk governance* (pp. 19–41). Dordrecht: Springer. https://doi.org/10.1007/978-94-017-9328-5_2
Renn, O., & Sellke, P. (2011). Risk, society and policy making: Risk governance in a complex world. *International Journal of Performability Engineering, 7,* 349.
Renn, O., Klinke, A., & Van Asselt, M. (2011). Coping with complexity, uncertainty and ambiguity in risk governance: A synthesis. *Ambio, 40,* 231–246.
Rittel, H. W., & Webber, M. M. (1973). 2.3 planning problems are wicked. *Polity, 4,* 155–169.
Rowe, W. D. (1977). *Anatomy of risk.* New York: Wiley.
Schneider, W., Körkel, J., & Weinert, F. E. (1989). Domain-specific knowledge and memory performance: A comparison of high-and low-aptitude children. *Journal of Educational Psychology, 81,* 306.
Shrader-Frechette, K. (1996). Methodological rules for four classes of scientific uncertainty. *Scientific uncertainty and environmental problem solving* (pp. 12–39). Cambridge, MA: Blackwell.

Slovic, P. (1999). Trust, emotion, sex, politics, and science: Surveying the risk-assessment battlefield. *Risk Analysis, 19,* 689–701.
Smith, D., & McCloskey, J. (2000). *History repeating itself? Risk management and society.* Dordrecht: Springer.
Spruijt, P., Knol, A. B., Vasileiadou, E., Devilee, J., Lebret, E., & Petersen, A. C. (2014). Roles of scientists as policy advisers on complex issues: A literature review. *Environmental Science & Policy, 40,* 16–25.
Stirling, A. (2003). Risk, uncertainty and precaution: Some instrumental implications from the social sciences. Negotiating change. In F. Berkhout (Ed.), *Negotiating Environmental Change: New Perspectives from Social Science* (pp. 33–76). Cheltenham: Edward Elgar.
Suleiman, E. N. (1977). The myth of technical expertise: Selection, organization, and leadership. *Comparative Politics, 10,* 137–158.
Thomas, J. W., & Grindle, M. S. (1990). After the decision: Implementing policy reforms in developing countries. *World Development, 18,* 1163–1181.
Titterton, M. (2004). *Risk and risk taking in health and social welfare.* London: Jessica Kingsley Publishers.
Tversky, A., & Kahneman, D. (1974). Judgment under uncertainty: Heuristics and biases. *Science, 185,* 1124–1131.
Underdal, A. (2010). Complexity and challenges of long-term environmental governance. *Global Environmental Change, 20,* 386–393.
Weber, E. P., & Khademian, A. M. (2008). Wicked problems, knowledge challenges, and collaborative capacity builders in network settings. *Public Administration Review, 68*(2), 334–349.
Ziman, J. (2002). *Real science: What it is and what it means.* Cambridge: Cambridge University Press.

CHAPTER 3

A Critique of the Social Amplification of Risk Framework from the Power Perspective

SOCIAL AMPLIFICATION OF RISK FRAMEWORK

The SARF (Kasperson et al. 1988), which relies on communication theory (Lasswell 1948; Shannon and Weaver 1949, 2015), illustrates how some risk events may become amplified (increase) or attenuated (decrease) and to this end shape behaviour. The SARF identifies two main mechanisms of 'amplification' in risk communication processes: the 'information mechanism' and the 'response mechanism' (Kasperson et al. 1988). The information mechanism comprises the sources, the channels and the transmission of the information. In this context, the volume of media coverage and information provided (including the event is framed), and the degree to which the information is disputed are central part of the information amplification mechanism (Kasperson and Kasperson 1996; Kasperson 2012). As such, the 'media' is seen as the main amplification station. The response mechanism on the other hand entails the behavioural response to the risk event. Critical factors identified to shape the response mechanism are heuristics, values, stigmatisation and social group relationships. Others are trust (Frewer 2003), culture (Masuda and Garvin 2006) and emotions (Morganstern 2016). Thus, the SARF views the information sources, channels, social/individual stations and institutional/social behaviour as key elements of social amplification.

The SARF uses the analogy of "dropping a stone in a pond" (Kasperson 2005, p. 78) where the ripple effect goes beyond the initial event. Such ripples could have secondary and tertiary impact and may be expressed in the form of financial losses, regulatory actions, increased/decreased institutional trust, stigmatisation and organisational change. This implies that the amplification occurs even in its transmission, in a way that may be linked with the issue-attention cycle. These signals are subject to distortion as they transition from one 'amplification' station to the other. Amplification stations may be individuals, interest groups, government and corporate organisations, policymakers, and pressure groups (Kasperson 2012).

The SARF has been tested empirically both in the US and the UK (Machlis and Rosa 1990; Renn et al. 1992; Freudenburg 1993; Kasperson and Kasperson 1996; Petts et al. 2001; Pidgeon and Barnett 2013). Some of these studies suggest that the framework is able to explain how certain factors shape behavioural responses to risk (Machlis and Rosa 1990; Freudenburg 1993; Renn et al. 1992; Burns et al. 1993; Kasperson 1992; Kasperson and Kasperson 1996). However, the secondary and tertiary ripple effects were identified to be more difficult to prove (Metz 1996; Pidgeon 1999). The framework has been recognised for making a genuine attempt at providing theoretical coherence to the field of risk communication and perception (Pidgeon and Henwood 2010), and is believed to offer a comprehensive multi-disciplinary structure that assists in identifying and categorising social phenomena, and in interpreting empirical data and theoretical insight (Renn 2011). Table 3.1 depicts the elements of the information and response mechanism of the SARF as adapted from the literature.

Table 3.1 Elements of social amplification

Information Mechanism	Response Mechanism
Communication processes—the *sources*, the *channels* and the *transmitters, receiver* of risk information.	Institutional and social behaviours
Media coverage	Heuristic and values
Volume of information provided	Social group relationships
Degree of information dispute	Signal values
Extent of dramatization	Stigmatisation
Symbolic connotation of information (including frames and discourse)	Trust
	Culture
	Emotions

Source: Adapted from extant literature

From Table 3.1 what can be observed in the information mechanism of the SARF is its emphasis on 'who' (i.e. sources, channels and transmitters), especially 'the media' and the nature of risk information itself such as media coverage and volume of information available. While this is valuable in shedding light on the amplification (or attenuation) processes to some extent, it ignores how underlying social and institutional factors shape elements of this information mechanism of the SARF. From this point of view, several weaknesses of the SARF are discernible (especially around the information mechanism that influences the response mechanism).

One apparent shortcoming of the framework is that it pays too little attention to underlying social or institutional factors that shape risk information and communication. For example, it ignores the roles of power and processes around expertise (discussed in Chap. 2) that shape how risk information is encoded, transmitted, decoded and fed back in risk communication. Besides, the amount of information provided by the media, for example, has been argued to be less relevant to whose interpretation of the risk is legitimised (Petts et al. 2001) and who controls the policy agendas (Majone 2006), deciding what risk issues enter into the risk arena for debate.

In addition, the translation of knowledge to use in risk communication via "expertise" (Pender 2001; Power 2007) and associated calculative practices points to other weaknesses of the SARF. Science and its experts are largely relied upon to make sense of the risk faced (Collingridge and Reeve 1986; Jasanoff 1996; Fischbacher-Smith 2012). Therefore, how expertise is brought to bear on risk has implications for how a risk signal is interpreted and accepted. Furthermore, the centrality of science and its experts in making sense of risk issues for other non-scientific stakeholder groups raises questions around the language in use and especially as risk communication involves an interactive process between experts and lay public.

Having stated this, it becomes essential that this book (which focuses on power and expertise) first attempts to address the critique of the SARF in other contexts for this framework to provide a useful and robust lens through which to understand how power and expertise shape risk communication. This is especially so in the policy context where the policy perspective taken on risk has far-reaching health, social and political consequences. Accordingly, one way to improve on the existing conceptualisation of the SARF is to:

(a) Examine how power shapes social amplification (or attenuation) processes in risk communication about public health and safety;
(b) Investigate how expertise shapes social amplification (or attenuation) processes in risk communication about public health and safety; and
(c) Draw on debates about communication and trust/credibility to emphasise the significance of communication and trust, in risk communication about public health and safety.

Communication has been highlighted as an important part of risk communication (Smith 1988, 1990) and trust is now generally accepted as a critical underpinning factor that shapes behavioural responses to risk information (Renn and Levine 1991; Kasperson et al. 1992; Slovic 1993; Casiday 2005; Earle and Siegrist 2008). This understanding will enable us to further develop existing understanding of the SARF and make it possible to draw out best practices for risk communication about public health and safety and its associated policy development (see Chap. 9).

Power in Risk Communication

Power in risk communication can be exercised at multiple phases of risk communication. These include: (a) within processes of risk communication (encoding, transmission, decoding and feedback); (b) in the nature of stakeholder relationship and (c) in the wider environmental context that shapes the arguments brought to bear on the debate by the different stakeholder groups. This review draws on early social theories of power to unpick how power is exercised at these three levels of risk communication. Here, we draw on the works of Lukes (1974), Giddens (1979), Foucault (1980) and Clegg (1989).

Three Dimensional View of Power

Steven (1974) presents a three-dimensional view of power. Moving from the obvious to the less obvious, it includes (a) decision-making power, (b) non-decision-making power and (c) ideological power. Decision-making power is a form of power exercised through decisions made, made explicit by the behavioral response that follows such decisions. The focus of this book is more about the less obvious forms of power. Hence, more attention is now given to the other two dimensions of power as proposed by Steven (1974).

Non-decision-making Power
The non-decision-making power akin to Bachrach and Baratz (1962) is less obvious than the first dimension. Here, power is exercised by deciding on what issues make it to the risk agenda and are included in the debate and discussion. Issues that make it to the agenda become amplified over other issues as they largely determine the nature of questions asked and whose expertise is called upon. A typical example is where the debate relating to identifying policy priorities and risk agendas is limited to a few elite groups and not subjected to wider public debates. The danger here is that policy priorities relating to risk may then become a reflection of only a few elite group members, and that risk concerns expressed by other groups (or larger sections of society) may be unwittingly neglected or consciously excluded from the risk agenda. In such a scenario, the significance of issues that make it onto the risk agenda is then enhanced (i.e. risk amplification) and the significance of those concerns that fail to make it to the policy agenda is reduced (i.e. risk attenuation).

Ideological Power
Ideological power is where people's perception, desire and acceptability of risk is shaped and influenced through everyday socialisation processes (e.g. through the media, expertise and control of information). For example, media communication allows certain views to be shared with the larger population and therefore have greater propensity to shape public risk discourse. Power may also be exercised through control of risk information and expertise (i.e. who, when, where and how much information is made available or concealed) that shapes the knowledge, arguments and burden of proof brought to bear on risk communication. For example, the then Prime Minister, Theresa May, was accused of concealing information from Parliament over the Northern Ireland backstop. Thus, she was found in contempt of Parliament for not revealing relevant information over the risk of Northern Ireland being split from the UK as exposed by Brexit legal documents. Those who do not have access to such 'classified' information, or to the necessary expertise, have to rely mostly on third-party sources for such information, which could be distorted, incomplete or costly to access by less resourced groups. The consequence of this is that

those with little or no access to such information will be at a disadvantage in mounting an effective challenge to the powerful interests dominating the risk arena (Adekola et al. 2017).

Agency and Structure
Giddens' (1979) agency and structure describes how patterns of social relationships define the structure and function of that social system, and highlights the importance of direct or diffuse stakeholder relationships. Such a relationship enables the exchange of information, opinion and views between stakeholders in a way that may inform societal practices and enhance the capabilities of these practices to effect change (Giddens 1979). Giddens' (1979) notion of power is important in risk communication for two reasons. First, patterns of social relationship allow exchange of views and opinion between certain groups that may disadvantage other perspectives, held by other groups not involved in the exchange. This social relationship may be direct or diffused (e.g. historical, evolving and institutionalised discourse). Second, these exchanges give rise to social structures and this societal (hierarchical) structure locates certain groups in positions of authoritative power (e.g. the expert/layman categorisation).

Resistance: Power as a Two-Way Process
Michel Foucault proposes a different view of power, suggesting that power may be expressed through 'resistance'.

> Where there is power, there is resistance… this resistance is never in a position of exteriority in relation to power. (Foucault 1978, p. 95)

As noted in the above quote, resistance as form of power is available wherever other forms of power exist (both obvious and hidden). This form of power is often displayed by less dominant or disadvantaged groups that feel their perspectives of risk are being ignored or suppressed. By means of resistance, less powerful groups challenge the dominant or legitimised risk perspective. Such action has been seen in the past to influence or change policy strategy taken to mitigate public health risk. A typical example of such resistive power being proven to be effective in the policy domain was the scenario where the Canadian government had to reduce the increase in cigarette tax (initially aimed at curtailing smoking). This reduction was due to a rise in the illegal sale of tobacco on the black market or because of easy access to cheap contraband tobacco products (Gabler and Katz 2010) that were equally, and perhaps more dangerously, detrimental to public health. The revision of such an increase in tax was based on the assumption that while tax discourages smoking, there is the potential that it will drive up the demand for contraband tobacco products (Gabler and Katz 2010). This form of power may tilt the balance of power at any stage of the communication process. In other words, risk debates and the exercise of power are not one-way—they occur between groups on different sides of the argument.

Giddens' (1979) and Foucault's (1980) perspectives of power are important because they both recognise that risk communication is a two-way process and that power relations exist between those involved in the communication process.

Circuit of Power

Clegg (1989) attempted to combine a number of these perspectives of power discussed here, which he developed in his circuit of power framework. Clegg (1989) describes how a combination of factors is defined by or creates domination or resistance in social relationships. These factors include social relations, agencies, standing conditions and outcomes; established rules and regulation of meaning and membership; exogenous environmental contingencies; and innovation in domination or resistance. One interesting feature of Clegg's (1989) circuit of power framework is the recognition of 'exogenous environmental contingencies', brought about by changes in the wider societal context. This is consistent with the fact that risk communication does not just exist in a vacuum but occurs within a wider societal context in cognisance of past events (or debates) (Fellenor et al. 2018), and the uncertainty of the future that shapes the arguments brought to bear on a risk debate (see Table 3.2).

COMMUNICATION AND TRUST IN RISK COMMUNICATION

Having considered how power shapes risk communication and amplification processes, we will now consider emerging debates around communication and trust in risk communication to emphasise the significance of communication (Smith 1988, 1990) and trust (Renn and Levine 1991; Kasperson et al. 1992; Slovic 1993; Casiday 2005; Earle and Siegrist 2008) in risk communication and the amplification (and attenuation) processes.

Table 3.2 Dimensions of power in risk communication adapted from the literature

Aspects of communication	Dimensions of power in risk communication	Manifestation mechanism	Questions
Communication process	Non-decision-making power	Control of risk agenda	Who decides (and makes decisions on) what issues make it to the policy agenda?
	Ideological power	Media Discourse Interpretation Framing	How is risk communicated, interpreted (or not) and by whom, for whom and to whom?
		Control of risk information	Where, when and how much is revealed or concealed?
Stakeholder relationship	Agency and structure	Social (professional) relationship	Who interacts with whom and how are views exchanged?
		Societal (hierarchical) structures	How is expertise defined, developed and trained?
	Tactics of domination and resistance	Policies, regulations, penalties, sanctions, petitions, open letters, strikes, boycotts, litigation	Was the intended action realised or not?
Environmental context	Historic events (debates), future uncertainties and the wider PESTEL factors	Uncertainties in the wider political, economic, social, technological, legal and ecological or environmental context Historic events/debate	What uncertainties within the wider environmental context (PESTEL) are important to the discussion? What is known, unknown, emerging or changing? What prior relevant debate has occurred?

Communication

Understanding the nature of risk faced by the public often involves communication between experts across multiple disciplines and between technical experts and other non-scientific groups. However, the way in which risk information is communicated is known to play a key role in influencing how that information is perceived or used by individuals (Kahneman and Tversky 1984). This raises important issues around the nature of language in use, in particular, the specific forms of language code or frames of reference used by the different stakeholders' groups engaged in the risk communication (Smith 1988). The language and frame of argument used in risk communication is important because it might prevent some groups within the public (e.g. lay public) from engaging in risk communication about public health and safety by serving as a barrier. It is also possible that the use of unfamiliar (or technical) terms may be 'intentional', designed to keep those who do not understand the codes outside of the debate and deny them the opportunity to make valuable contributions to risk communication processes (Adekola et al. 2017).

Trust

Trust is believed to affect judgement of risk and benefit, and risk acceptability (Siegrist et al. 2003), and has been long recognised in the literature as a key element in risk communication (Kasperson et al. 1992; Löfstedt and Horlick-Jones 1999; Frewer 2003). The effect of trust in risk communication can be seen in how the lay public often defer sense making to experts, such that it makes them immediately vulnerable to the interpretations of experts in their understanding of risk. This vulnerability paradigm has been highlighted in several definitions of trust. For example, Mayer et al. (1995) and Kjærnes et al. (2007) describe trust as the 'willingness' to be vulnerable to the decisions and actions of another, where the trustee hopes to be considered and protected. Information about risk from a trusted source is argued to contribute to the way the receiver perceives and responds to the received information (Frewer et al. 2003). Flynn et al. (1992) explain that the more trustworthy a source (all other factors being equal), the more the information from this source will resonate with the audience. The opposite holds when the source of information is not trusted.

Cacioppo and Petty (1984) identify two routes by which a risk message can be decoded: the central route and the peripheral route. Trust plays a key role in determining which route is used in decoding the meaning inherent in the risk information received. The central route is where the receiver of risk information carries out an intense scrutiny of the risk information received. Here, external clues do not influence how the information is processed; the receiver carries out in-depth analyses of the risk information in a way that may serve either to reassure the decoder, attenuating risk concern, or to amplify the risk, especially where uncertainties or gaps in the knowledge are high. The peripheral route utilises those external clues, for example, the credibility of the source of information, an expert or known source, the timing and how the message is codified. These external cues allow the receptor of the risk information to make simple inferences and judgements about the merits of its content without any elaborate or in-depth processing. The danger here is that errors, distortion and gaps in risk messages are received without scrutiny. This may lead to a false perception of risk that may either amplify or attenuate the perspectives taken on risk. Insight from the work of Cacioppo and Petty (1984) suggests that the central route in decoding risk information is more likely to be used where there is absence of trust and credibility in the information source. The peripheral route is most likely to be used in situations of trust and credibility.

Trust also has implications for the nature of the feedback, which is recognised as essential for effective communication (Shannon 1961). Trust is believed to encourage openness, transparency, responsiveness and a willingness to consult with one another (Fischbacher-Smith et al. 2010). A receiver who trusts the sender of the message is likely to be more inclined to have an honest conversation than with a source that is mistrusted (Gabarro 1978). This is because where trust exists, it is more probable to share difficult feelings and concerns and this can be dealt with appropriately. This reduces the pressure towards increased risk concern created by other factors. Fischbacher-Smith et al. (2010) argue that where the qualities of openness, transparency, responsiveness and willingness to consult with one another are lacking, there is greater possibility of risk intensification.

The literature described in this chapter highlights the significance of how power, expertise, communication and trust shape the processes of amplification (and attenuation) in risk communication. These four themes have been conceptualised into a framework, the PERC framework (Adekola et al. 2018), which explains the risk amplification (or attenuation) processes in the policy domain.

THE POLICY EVALUATION RISK COMMUNICATION (PERC) FRAMEWORK

According to Adekola et al. (2018), power, expertise, communication and trust are key factors that influence policy discussions about risk in the amplification (or attenuation) processes. This is especially the case where there is weak scientific evidence that allows multiple perspectives and strong power dynamics to thrive. The PERC framework assumes that the 'social amplification (or attenuation) of risk' is the core driver that shapes how an argument about risk within a set of arguments becomes amplified in the policy domain (Fig. 3.1).

The core argument of the PERC framework is that public debates are shaped by multiple levels of interaction of power and expertise that can enhance or inhibit the perspective of some public groups in a public debate. These multiple levels of interaction of power and expertise create but can also destroy trust and privilege in the scientific understanding of risk over other perspectives. The consequence of this is that it causes a power disequilibrium in risk debates such that an argument within a set of

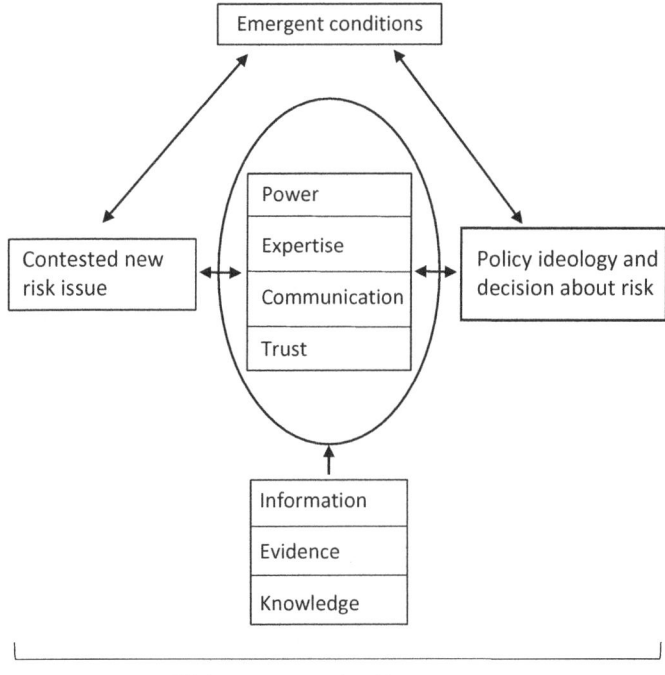

Fig. 3.1 Policy Evaluation Risk Communication (PERC) framework. (Source: Adekola et al. 2018)

risk arguments could dominate over other legitimate perspectives. It is on this basis that this book adopts the PERC framework as a means of unpicking and evidencing how power and expertise shape debates about public health and safety. The next three chapters (4, 5 and 6) examine the cases of the smoking, MMR vaccine and sugar debates in the UK. These cases will then be analysed through the PERC framework (in Chap. 7) to highlight how power (see Chap. 3) and expertise (see Chap. 2) shape risk communication about public health and safety.

References

Adekola, J., Fischbacher-Smith, M., Fischbacher-Smith, D., & Adekola, O. (2017). Health risks from environmental degradation in the Niger Delta, Nigeria. *Environment and Planning C: Politics and Space, 35,* 334–354.

Adekola, J., Fischbacher-Smith, D., & Fischbacher-Smith, M. (2018). Light me up: Power and expertise in risk communication and policy-making in the e-cigarette health debates. *Journal of Risk Research,* 1–15.

Bachrach, P., & Baratz, M. S. (1962). Two faces of power. *American Political Science Review, 56,* 947–952.

Burns, W. J., Slovic, P., Kasperson, R. E., Kasperson, J. X., Renn, O., & Emani, S. (1993). Incorporating structural models into research on the social amplification of risk: Implications for theory construction and decision making. *Risk Analysis, 13,* 611–623.

Cacioppo, J. T., & Petty, R. E. (1984). The elaboration likelihood model of persuasion. *ACR North American Advances.*

Casiday, R. E. (2005). *Risk conceptualisations, trust and decision-making in the face of contradictory information: The case of MMR.* Durham: Durham University.

Clegg, S. R. (1989). *Frameworks of power.* London: Sage.

Collingridge, D., & Reeve, C. (1986). *Science speaks to power: The role of experts in policy making.* London: Pinter.

Earle, T., & Siegrist, M. (2008). Trust, confidence and cooperation model: A framework for understanding the relation between trust and risk perception. *International Journal of Global Environmental Issues, 8,* 17–29.

Fellenor, J., Barnett, J., Potter, C., Urquhart, J., Mumford, J., & Quine, C. P. (2018). Ash dieback and other tree pests and pathogens: Dispersed risk events and the social amplification of risk framework. *Journal of Risk Research,* 1–33.

Fischbacher-Smith, D. (2012). Getting pandas to breed: Paradigm blindness and the policy space for risk prevention, mitigation and management. *Risk Management, 14,* 177–201.

Fischbacher-Smith, D., Irwin, A., & Fischbacher-Smith, M. (2010). Bringing light to the shadows and shadows to the light: Risk, risk management, and risk communication. In P. Bennet, K. Calman, S. Curtis, & D. Fischbacher-Smith (Eds.), *Risk communication and public health* (pp. 23–38). Oxford University Press: Oxford. https://doi.org/10.1093/acprof:oso/9780199562848.003.02. ISBN 9780199562848.

Flynn, J., Burns, W., Mertz, C. K., & Slovic, P. (1992). Trust as a determinant of opposition to a high-level radioactive waste repository: Analysis of a structural model. *Risk analysis, 12*(3), 417–429.

Foucault, M. (1978). *The history of sexuality: Volume I. An Introduction.* New York: Vintage.

Foucault, M. (1980). *Power/knowledge: Selected interviews and other writings, 1972–1977.* Pantheon.

Freudenburg, W. R. (1993). Risk and recreancy: Weber, the division of labor, and the rationality of risk perceptions. *Social Forces, 71,* 909–932.

Frewer, L. J. (2003). *Trust, transparency, and social context: Implications for social amplification of risk.* Cambridge: Cambridge University Press.

Frewer, L. J., Scholderer, J., & Bredahl, L. (2003). Communicating about the risks and benefits of genetically modified foods: The mediating role of trust. *Risk Analysis, 23,* 1117–1133.

Gabarro, J. J. (1978). The development of trust, influence, and expectations. In *Interpersonal behavior: Communication and understanding in relationships* (pp. 290–303). Englewood Cliffs: Prentice-Hall.

Gabler, N., & Katz, D. (2010). *Contraband tobacco in Canada: Tax policies and black market incentives.* Vancouver: Fraser Institute.

Giddens, A. (1979). Agency, structure. In *Central problems in social theory* (pp. 49–95). London: Palgrave.

Jasanoff, S. (1996). Beyond epistemology: Relativism and engagement in the politics of science. *Social Studies of Science, 26,* 393–418.

Kahneman, D., & Tversky, A. (1984). Choices, values, and frames. *American Psychologist, 39,* 341.

Kasperson, R. E. (1992). *The social amplification of risk: Progress in developing an integrative framework in social theories of risk.* Santa Barbara: Praeger.

Kasperson, R. E. (2005). *Social contours of risk: Publics, risk communication and the social amplification of risk.* London: Earthscan.

Kasperson, R. E. (2012). *Social contours of risk: Volume I: Publics, risk communication and the social.* London: Routledge.

Kasperson, R. E., & Kasperson, J. X. (1996). The social amplification and attenuation of risk. In *The Annals of the American Academy of Political and Social Science* (pp. 95–105). Thousand Oaks: Sage. https://journals.sagepub.com/doi/abs/10.1177/0002716296545001010

Kasperson, R. E., Renn, O., Slovic, P., Brown, H. S., Emel, J., Goble, R., Kasperson, J. X., & Ratick, S. (1988). The social amplification of risk: A conceptual framework. *Risk Analysis, 8*, 177–187.

Kasperson, R. E., Golding, D., & Tuler, S. (1992). Social distrust as a factor in siting hazardous facilities and communicating risks. *Journal of Social Issues, 48*, 161–187.

Kjærnes, U., Harvey, M., & Warde, A. (2007). *Trust in food: A comparative and institutional analysis*. Basingstoke: Palgrave Macmillan.

Lasswell, H. D. (1948). The structure and function of communication in society. *The Communication of Ideas, 37*, 215–228.

Löfstedt, R. E., & Horlick-Jones, T. (1999). Environmental regulation in the UK: Politics, institutional change and public trust. In *Social trust and the management of risk* (pp. 73–88). London: Earthscan.

Lukes, S. (1974). *Power: A radical view*. London: Macmillan.

Machlis, G. E., & Rosa, E. A. (1990). Desired risk: Broadening the social amplification of risk Framework. *Risk Analysis, 10*, 161–168.

Majone, G. (2006). *Agenda setting*. Oxford/New York: Oxford University Press.

Masuda, J. R., & Garvin, T. (2006). Place, culture, and the social amplification of risk. *Risk Analysis, 26*, 437–454.

Mayer, R. C., Davis, J. H., & Schoorman, F. D. (1995). An integrative model of organizational trust. *Academy of Management Review, 20*, 709–734.

Metz, W. C. (1996). Historical application of a social amplification of risk model: Economic impacts of risk events at nuclear weapons facilities. *Risk Analysis, 16*, 185–193.

Morganstern, A. (2016). *The interaction of emotion and gender on the social amplification of risk: Why Twitter?* Eugene: University of Oregon.

Pender, S. (2001). Managing incomplete knowledge: Why risk management is not sufficient. *International Journal of Project Management, 19*, 79–87.

Petts, J., Horlick-Jones, T., Murdock, G., Hargreaves, D., McLachlan, S., & Lofstedt, R. (2001). *Social amplification of risk: The media and the public*. Sudbury: HSE Books.

Pidgeon, N. (1999). Risk communication and the social amplification of risk: Theory, evidence and policy implications. *Risk Decision and Policy, 4*, 145–159.

Pidgeon, N., & Barnett, J. (2013). *Chalara and the social amplification of risk*. London: Department for Environment, Food and Rural Affairs.

Pidgeon, N., & Henwood, K. (2010). The social amplification of risk framework (SARF): Theory, critiques, and policy implications. In P. Bennett, K. Calman, S. Curtis, & D. Fischbacher-Smith (Eds.), *Risk communication and public health* (2nd ed.). Oxford: Oxford University Press.

Power, M. (2007). *Organised uncertainty*. Oxford: Oxford University Press.

Renn, O. (2011). The social amplification/attenuation of risk framework: Application to climate change. *Wiley Interdisciplinary Reviews: Climate Change, 2*, 154–169.

Renn, O., & Levine, D. (1991). Credibility and trust in risk communication. In *Communicating risks to the public* (pp. 175–217). Dordrecht: Springer.

Renn, O., Burns, W. J., Kasperson, J. X., Kasperson, R. E., & Slovic, P. (1992). The social amplification of risk: Theoretical foundations and empirical applications. *Journal of Social Issues, 48*, 137–160.

Shannon, C. E. (1961). Two-way communication channels. In *Proceedings of 4th Berkeley symposium on mathematical statistics and probability, 1961, USA* (pp. 611–644). Berkeley: Statistical Laboratory of the University of California.

Shannon, C. E., & Weaver, W. (1949). *The mathematical theory of communication*. Urbana: University of Illinois Press.

Shannon, C. E., & Weaver, W. (2015). *The mathematical theory of communication*. Urbana: University of Illinois Press.

Siegrist, M., Earle, T. C., & Gutscher, H. (2003). Test of a trust and confidence model in the applied context of electromagnetic field (EMF) risks. *Risk Analysis, 23*, 705–716.

Slovic, P. (1993). Perceived risk, trust, and democracy. *Risk Analysis, 13*, 675–682.

Smith, D. (1988). *Corporate power, risk assessment and the control of major hazards: A study of Canvey Island and Ellesmere Port*. Manchester: University of Manchester.

Smith, D. (1990). *Corporate power, risk assessment and the control of major hazards: A study of Canvey Island and Ellesmere Port*. PhD dissertation, University of Manchester.

Steven, L. (1974). *Power: A radical view*. London/New York: Macmillan.

CHAPTER 4

The UK Smoking Debate

THE SMOKING DEBATE (1950 TO 1955)

In September 1950, the first large-scale epidemiological study by Doll and Hill (1950) suggested a 'real association' between smoking tobacco and cancer, especially of the lungs. Doll and Hill (1950) concluded that smoking was linked to lung cancer after examining over 1300 men with this type of cancer, and found that 99.5% of them smoked tobacco cigarettes. The research examined around 5000 hospital patients in UK hospitals and established that a statistical relationship does indeed exist, thus linking smoking tobacco and lung cancer (Doll and Hill 1950). Earlier that year, two studies (Wynder and Graham 1950; Levin et al. 1950) came to similar conclusions that there was potentially a link between the two. The initial reaction to Doll and Hill's (1950) research linking smoking to lung cancer was received with scepticism within both the scientific and medical community (Lopez 1999). Smoking at this point was considered a natural and sophisticated behaviour and was allowed everywhere including in offices, pubs, restaurants, cinemas and all transport systems (Peto et al. 2000).

Six months after Doll and Hill's (1950) publication, two key government advisory groups, the Central Health Services Committee (CHSC) and the Standing Advisory Committee on Cancer and Radiotherapy (SACCR), accepted Doll and Hill's findings and advised the government to accept the emerging evidence linking smoking tobacco and lung cancer (CHSC and SACCR 1951). According to the group,

Professor Bradford Hill and Dr Doll are satisfied that the case against smoking as such is proven. (CHSC and SACCR 1951)

This acceptance of Doll and Hill's conclusion is evidence of the weight given to technical expertise within the policy domain. It also shows the significance of such a relationship between policymakers and technical experts (stakeholders) in unifying their risk discourse in the policy domain. Following this initial publication, Doll and Hill extended their investigation (which had initially been limited to the London area) to Bristol, Cambridge, Leeds and Newcastle-upon-Tyne (Doll and Hill 1952). This second study reached a similar conclusion to the first, providing further statistical evidence to prove the relationship between smoking tobacco and lung cancer. However, in February of 1953, the CHSC received a report from Imperial Tobacco Statistical Department which seemed to be an attempt to disprove Doll and Hill's findings (Teague 1953). In a statement directed to shareholders, the Chairman of Imperial Tobacco says,

> If it should ever be proved that there exists something harmful in tobacco, even in the minutest quantities, which could conceivably make smoking one of the causes of this disease [cancer], we should, I hope, be the first to take steps to eliminate it. (Chairman of Imperial Tobacco Statement 1953)

The above statement from the representative of the Imperial Tobacco Statistical Department suggests that the company understood the importance of trust in shaping the risk debate as they demanded they should be trusted; this is evidenced by the statement: "if it should ever be proved that there exists something harmful in tobacco... [They] will be the first to act ...." Later that year, the Chief Medical Officer at the Ministry of Health went further to set up a statistical panel to look at the relationship between smoking tobacco and cancer. This analysis also confirmed that there was a statistical connection between the two. The Ministry of Health stated that

> We are therefore of the opinion that the main conclusion reached by Doll and Hill, that there is a real association between smoking tobacco and cancer of the lung, is firmly established. (Statistical Panel and MoH Report 1953, cited in Pollock 1999)

At this point, the nature of evidence was still statistical in nature. The first ever study to show a biological link between smoking tobacco and lung cancer was published in December of 1953. The research found that cigarette tar was painted on the backs of mice led to the growth of tumours over time (Wynder et al. 1953). In March of 1955, the CHSC advised the Minister for Health to take appropriate action in informing the public that tobacco and heavy smoking were dangerous to health (CHSC and SACCR 1956). They asserted that

> It must be regarded as established that there is a relationship between smoking tobacco and cancer of the lung. (CHSC and SACCR 1953)

In January of 1954, the UK Health Minister accepted the link between smoking tobacco and lung cancer, while being cautious around the fact that evidence of how smoking is linked to lung cancer remains weak. In a memo written to the Cabinet Home Affairs Committee, the minister stated that

> [I have] come to the conclusion that the statistical evidence does point to a causal relationship between tobacco smoking tobacco and cancer of the lung, but that there are important qualifications. There is no precise evidence of how tobacco smoking causes cancer of the lung or indeed of the extent to which one causes the other. (Minister of Health 1954, cited in WHO 2016)

As more evidence continued to show a link between smoking tobacco and lung cancer (Hammond and Horn 1954; Doll and Hill 1954), tobacco manufacturers in the UK, including leading names such as British American Tobacco (BAT), Gallaher and Imperial, denied that there was a link between smoking tobacco and lung cancer. They argued that more biological evidence would be needed before any such assertions could be made. The industry offered £250,000 to aid the Medical Research Council (MRC) research and expressed in a statement that

> This can only be the case when medical science is able to provide a causal proof to the claim. (Statement Issued by the Group of Leading Tobacco Manufacturers 1954, cited in Libal 2014)

Despite the strong acknowledgement of the results of Doll and Hill and publications by the medical and scientific community and public health experts at this point, the evolving events suggest that no immediate action was taken by the UK government to mitigate the dangers of smoking to public health. Aside from the fact that smoking was considered a normal thing to do in the 1950s, the initial response by the government (inactivity) was also influenced by a number of situational factors during this period. This includes the role played by the industry in shaping the debate and the economic significance of tobacco to the UK government (in terms of jobs and tax contributions). Tobacco companies in the UK paid high taxes and were a major source of employment in Britain. Therefore, the government may not have wanted to interfere with this (at least until there was an alternative source of income and employment). It is possible that for economic reasons, the government ignored the excesses of tobacco companies and the dangers these posed to public health. In addition, policymakers were concerned about the nature of existing evidence, as can be seen above in the Minister of Health's statement in 1954. Advising a change to such ingrained societal behaviour would require evidence and communication sustained over a decent period of time to achieve the desired behavioural goal.

THE SMOKING DEBATE (1956 AND 1965)

The period between 1956 and 1965 saw greater weight of evolving scientific evidence giving credence to the claim that smoking is linked to lung cancer (Schwartz and Denoix 1957; Stocks 1958; Haenszel et al. 1958; Dorn 1959; Doll et al. 1957; Hilding 1956; Kotin et al. 1956; Auerbach et al. 1957; Chang 1957; Leuchtenberger et al. 1958; Bock and Moore 1959; Engelbreth-Holm and Ahlmann 1957; Gellhorn 1958; Orris et al. 1958; Lyons and Johnston 1957; Van Duuren 1958; Wynder and Wright 1957; Wynder et al. 1958), although most studies remained statistical. The absence or near absence of any causal proof (biological or experimental evidence) may be due to the fact that it is difficult and costly in terms of time and financial resources to generate, or even because it was 'intentionally' avoided, since causal proof would be too damaging for the tobacco industry. This is perhaps one reason why representatives of the industry were fiercely engaged in undermining the technical case linking smoking tobacco and lung cancer. They argued that more research was needed before any causal association or claim could be established.

The evolving events within this period shows that in February of 1956, a study published by Dr. Ernest Wynder and his colleagues found a link between the risk of developing larynx cancer and an increase in the amount of smoke consumed (Wynder et al. 1958). In a letter to Sir John Hawton,

Ministry of Health, the tobacco industry reassured the government of their commitment to public health:

> "There is no proof at all that smoking causes cancer of the lung and much to suggest that it cannot be the cause" (Partridge 1956) ... "We would regard it an elementary duty and responsibility to leave nothing undone that we can do to secure the eradication of anything in tobacco which is found to be harmful to health." (Partridge 1956)

The above statement again is an indication of the demand for public trust by representatives of the tobacco industry.

In May of 1956, Mr. Turton, the Minister of Health, stated that the government should take a precautionary stance on tobacco control. In the House of Commons, he explained that

> Two known cancer-causing agents have been identified in tobacco smoke, but whether they have a direct role in producing cancer of the lung, and if so what, has not been proved. (Turton 1956, cited in BBC News 1956)

He did, however, acknowledge that "mortality from cancer of the lung is twenty times greater amongst heavy smokers than amongst non-smokers" (Turton, 1956, cited in BBC news 1956).

However, despite the seeming consensus as noted above and a push by key government officials that smoking was statistically associated with lung cancer, the evolving events suggest that no immediate or considerable action was taken by the government at this point. In August of 1956, British tobacco manufacturers formed a committee known as the Tobacco Manufacturers' Standing Committee (TMSC) (Glantz et al. 1996). The establishment of TMSC increased the industry's capacity to exercise stronger power over scientific evidence and its interpretation. In June of 1957, the MRC published a five-year report, "Tobacco Smoking and Lung Cancer". The report, which was accepted by the Minister of Health, links the increase in deaths from lung cancer with smoking, especially cigarettes. The report states that

> The most reasonable interpretation of scientific evidence is that the relationship is one of direct cause and effect... The identification of several carcinogenic substances in tobacco smoke provides a rational basis for such a causal relationship. (MRC Report 1957)

In his statement, the minister equated this statistical evidence with causal proof. However, representatives of the tobacco industry immediately challenged his contention. For instance, a statement from a representative of TMSC reads that

> It has not been established with any certainty whether and to what extent there may be a causal relationship between smoking tobacco and cancer of the lung. At this stage any conclusions are a matter of opinion. (The Guardian 2010)

In July of 1958, the evolution of events suggests that another argument has emerged. Fisher (1958) suggested that an individual's 'genes' might predispose them to smoking tobacco and contracting cancer. Fisher, who later became a consultant for TMSC, argued that the smoking causal argument was unproven. He noted that the genetic argument was more plausible as supported by new evidence, a result of an inquiry into the smoking habits of adult male twin pairs on their list (Fisher 1958). Fisher in his study examined 51 monozygotic twins (identical) and 31 dizygotic twins (fraternal) from Tubingen, Frankfurt and Berlin (Fisher 1959). He concluded that genotype does have an effect on smoking behaviour and on smoking habits adopted. The study noted that different genotype groups would be different in terms of incidence of cancer.

In discrediting Doll and Hill's argument, Fisher concentrated on the negative correlation between inhaling cigarette smoke and lung cancer in their 1950 study. He questioned the MRC conclusions of Doll and Hill's (1950) study, arguing that they were jumping from the observation of an association to the conclusion of a causal relationship. To emphasise the point, Fisher noted that if the MRC were to jump to a conclusion on the case of inhaling cigarette smoke, it would lead to a conclusion that cigarettes cause cancer but that inhaling cigarette smoke prevents it. A further study also emerged in support of the genetic argument: in 1960, Eysenck criticised the causal argument, noting that smoking has ameliorating effects with respect to lung cancer (Eysenck et al. 1960).

Royal College of Physicians (RCP) First Report

The Royal College of Physicians (RCP) research committee looked into smoking and atmospheric pollution in relation to carcinoma of the lungs and other diseases, and published its first report in March of 1962. The report, entitled "Smoking and Health", argued that cigarette smoking causes cancer and bronchitis (RCP Report 1962) and pointed out that smoking is a cause of the rise in cancer cases. The report rated the number of deaths related to lung cancer as higher in the UK than in any other country in the world, and that lung cancer exposes people to the risk of developing chronic bronchitis and coronary heart disease, particularly in early middle age. The report recommended that there should be strict regulation of tobacco sale and advertisement, introduction of taxes to curb smoking, and further restriction on selling tobacco to those who are underage. There was also a recommendation to curb smoking in public spaces. This RCP recommendation became the core of tobacco control policies worldwide over the next 60 years (RCP Report 1992) and the origin of many of the arguments that arose within the tobacco debate.

The RCP report received widespread publicity on the day of its publication, and there was a press conference to disseminate the findings, a technique used to announce scientific conclusions of high interest to the general public. At the time of this report, around 70% and 40% of men and women respectively in the UK smoked tobacco cigarette. Smoking was allowed in all public spaces including schools, workplaces, hospitals and travel systems. BBC archive footage on the Tonight programme, which was aired on the night of the publication, captured public opinion on the suggestion that tobacco causes lung cancer (Hughes 2012). One man who smoked between 20 and 25 cigarettes per day stated,

> Quite honestly, I think that the end of one's life is probably more in the hands of almighty God you know, than in my own hands or the hands of the tobacco manufacturers.

Another interviewee said,

> I think so, yes. If I'm going to die, I'm going to die, so I might as well enjoy life as it is now.

A third interviewee mentioned how she tried to quit but was not able to manage beyond two days. Another thought that if she didn't smoke she would be miserable. This suggests a deep-rooted smoking culture and societal acceptance of smoking in the 1950s and 1960s. In response to the RCP report, G.F. Todd of Imperial tobacco stated that

> there is no denial of the almost certain relationship between smoking tobacco and cancer of the lung although it is possible this is done in the light to confuse the issue. (G.F. Todd, Comments on the RCP Report 1962)

Days after the RCP report, John Partridge, an executive of Imperial Tobacco, was featured on the BBC's Panorama programme (Libal 2014). He suggested that the RCP report expressed an "unbalanced picture" of existing knowledge, and uncertainties regarding smoking.

> I do not believe that you will stop the people of this country from smoking … they know the odds are heavily against their coming to any real harm from it. (cited in Libal 2014)

The Chairman of the Imperial Tobacco Company, R W S Clark, in an address to the annual general meeting, debunked the idea that commercial interest was the main motivation for the position of the industry on statistical evidence suggesting a link between smoking and other diseases. The Chairman, seeking public trust, said that

> It has been said or implied in a number of quarters that the position taken up by the manufacturers is heavily biased by the fact our commercial interests are involved. I want to say quite categorically that any such imputation is completely unjustified and unfair. It is, of course, self-evident that the industry's commercial interests are involved, but the tobacco manufacturers also fully recognise their responsibility to the public. (Clarke 1962)

During the BAT annual research conference, Sir Charles Ellis suggested that the interpretation given to statistical links between smoking tobacco and lung cancer was one with an "emotional gloss":

> We who have been immersed in the subject for many years know that this report produced no new fact, produced no new arguments, indeed, except for the contribution of an emotional gloss, left the subject untouched. We know only too well that there are no conclusive proofs; that there are few, if any, cold scientific facts. However emotional conclusions cannot be disregarded. (McCormick 1962)

In May of 1964, Doll and Hill published their third study on smoking tobacco and cancer, extending their study to all parts of Britain. They conducted a survey on "Mortality in Relation to Smoking: Ten Years' Observations of British Doctors" (Doll and Hill 1964). Three years earlier, the researchers had sent a short survey to 59,600 members of the public registered on the British Medical Register and residing in the UK. The study found that 50% of the UK's doctors who smoked had given up between 1951 and 1964. They also found a significant decline in incidences of cancer among those who stopped smoking when compared to those who did not (Doll and Hill 1964).

After much pressure (mainly from the Standing Medical Advisory Committee, the CHSC, many MPs and the Chief Medical Officers at the Ministry of Health) on the government to enforce tobacco control, the first government response came in 1965. The UK government, after consultation with the Independent Television Authority, banned television advertising of tobacco products under the Television Act, 1964 (ash.org.uk).

The Smoking Risk Debate (between 1966 and 1998)

The period between 1966 and 1998 is the longest period under assessment in this case study. This is because the evolution of events suggests that politicians and government public health departments had formed an ideology in which smoking was considered dangerous to health (see above paragraph). However, there was yet to be any concrete action from the government in mitigating the risks of smoking. The period between 1966 and 1998 saw a ban on tobacco advertisement, greater protection of young children and a change of voluntary agreement governance (which was circumvented in some instances (Smith 1982)) to legally binding rules in relation to advertising and selling tobacco cigarettes.

In January of 1971, the Royal College of Physicians published another report titled "Smoking and Health Now". The number of deaths associated with smoking was described as a present-day "'holocaust' that is shortening the life of the public" (RCP Report 1971).

The report also suggested a clear socio-economic divide in giving up smoking. Those in 'professional classes' (e.g. doctors) were found to be smoking less; however, people in the low-wage and manual groups continued in their smoking behaviour. This suggested that there are distributive inequalities associated with the understanding of risk with those in poorer sections of society suffering the most from impact of errors in the understanding of risk. Following this publication, RCP set up Action on Smoking and Health (ASH). Its remit was to de-glamourise the act of smoking in society and to create public awareness about the dangers of smoking. In March of 1971, the Secretary of State for Health, Sir Keith Joseph, restated the government's position on control of tobacco, which was one of voluntary agreement with the tobacco industry (ash.org.uk).

In April of 1971, a voluntary agreement, the first of its kind, was proposed between the government and the tobacco industry. The arrangement included providing warnings on cigarette packs and in all forms of media adverts. There was also the agreement to invent new technologies to reduce the dangers of smoking (ash.org.uk). In May of the same year, cigarette advertisements on radio were also banned in the UK.

In January of 1972, 132 MPs in the House of Commons voted to ban cigarette advertising; 73 were against this ban (ash.org.uk). This signified political support for a ban on tobacco advertising and was essential at this point because advertisements for tobacco would be counter-productive to the government strategy of raising public awareness on the dangers of smoking. The existing voluntary agreement was also extended and this included 'health hints' on packets of cigarettes, and brand advertisements at sporting events and on advertisements sent through the post. In May of 1972, in a press release issued by the Tobacco Institute, Richard Dobson, who was to become Chairman of BAT, says,

> It's hard to argue that filling your lungs with smoke can be actually good for you. But surely it is a question of moderation and I do sincerely believe that the tobacco industry, in total, does more good than harm. (ash.org.uk)

By 1975, the Harrogate research facility of the UK tobacco industry was closed down (RJ Reynolds Research Department 1976, cited in WHO 2016). In March, Sir John Partridge from Imperial expressed the opinion that

> As a company we do not make, indeed we are not qualified to make, medical judgements. We are therefore not in a position either to accept or to reject statements made by the Minister of Health.

The above statement suggests that the industry was tempering its attack on the technical case linking smoking tobacco and lung cancer, now accepted by politicians and departments of government. In January of 1977, a TV campaign was launched by the Health Education Council (HEC) with a focus on protecting the interests of non-smokers and women. In April of the same year, a paper on "Smoking and Health: the Effect on Marketing" was written by P. L Short, from BAT. This paper commented on the benefits of smoking and found a direct relationship between smoking and improvement in certain behaviours of individual 'subjects'.

In April of 1980, Patrick Sheehy, former chairperson of BAT, wrote to BBC Panorama about the continuing smoking controversy, saying that

> Scientists are [by] no means unanimous regarding smoking and health issues … we would therefore ask you to ensure that the programme disassociates the views of the scientist in question [Dr Jim Green] from those of this company by making an appropriate statement to this effect in the programme. (P. Sheehy, Letter to the BBC 1980)

BBC Panorama revealed that the chairperson of the Tobacco Advisory Council was also on the UK Sports Council. It also revealed how the industry had refused to publicly acknowledge that smoking was dangerous and potentially a killer. On the programme, Dr. Green, now retired from BAT, admitted that smoking played a significant role in the development of lung cancer. Nevertheless, associates of the tobacco industry continued to dispel the relationship between smoking and lung cancer.

In November of 1984, the RCP report "Smoking still kills" was published. It urged the government to do more to curb the dangers of tobacco (Taylor 1984). That month an R. J. Reynolds Tobacco Company advertisement proclaimed that

> It has been stated so often that smoking causes cancer, it's no wonder most people believe this is an established fact. But, in fact, it is nothing of the kind. The truth is that almost three decades of research have failed to produce scientific proof for this claim … in our opinion, the issue of smoking tobacco and cancer of the lung is not a closed case. It's an open controversy. (Report of Special Master 1998)

In March of 1982, the Presidents of the UK's eight Royal Colleges of Medicine in a letter to the UK government stated that deaths and disability associated with tobacco could easily be prevented (Smith 1982). The letter in the *British Medical Journal* (*BMJ*) highlighted concerns of sports sponsorship by tobacco interests and recommended a total ban on sports sponsorship (Smith 1982). That same month, the highest percentage rise since 1947 in cigarette tax was implemented. The 14 pence tax rise was passed on to smokers with the aim of discouraging them from smoking by increasing the price.

By October of 1982, a new voluntary agreement with the tobacco industry to regulate advertising and promotion was announced by the government. Its provisions included display of health warnings on cigarette parks and regulation of advertisements at point of sale (ash.org.uk). The industry agreed to reduce poster and cinema advertisements by almost 50% and offered to continue to fund health-related research. The agreement received widespread criticism from both the public and media (ash.org.uk). In March of 1984, a study entitled "The Smoke Ring" revealed how the tobacco industry had planned to remain in business despite widespread evidence of the health dangers of its product (Taylor 1985). A study published the following year received massive publicity as BBC Panorama featured it on the day of its publication (Taylor 1985).

In January of 1985, churches and health organisations were drawn into the controversy and were embarrassed after the British Medical Association (BMA)'s report showed that they had investments in tobacco companies (ash.org.uk). A study by Alderson et al. (1985) further implicated tobacco smoking by discovering reduced cases of lung cancer amongst ex-smokers. Communicating the scientific underpinnings of the smoking risk remained relevant in this debate. In this case, the HEC launched a campaign targeted at women where the argument was framed by stating that lung cancer kills as many women as breast cancer. Breast cancer is of course a major cause of death among women.

In November of 1985, a report by the HEC revealed that UK television broadcast over 330 hours of tobacco-sponsored programmes a year Turner (1987). In December, George Foulkes, Labour MP, introduced a Private Member's Bill designed to urge employers to increase non-smoking places or facilities in the workplace (ash.org.uk). In December of the same year, the *BMJ* condemned the Health Promotion Research Trust funded by the tobacco industry as "taking money from the Devil". It was suggested that sponsored research often favours the sponsors (ash.org.uk). In January of 1986, the HEC announced it would withhold grants from researchers and academics who receive funds from the tobacco industry-supported Health Promotion Research Trust (ash.org.uk).

Flurry of Events

In April, the UK government passed the "Protection of Children (Tobacco) Act" making it illegal for to sell tobacco to anyone under the age of 16 years. In February of 1987, Independent Television (ITV) stopped the transmission of all tobacco-sponsored sports events on its programmes (BBC 2009). In September, the European Commission launched "Europe Against Cancer", a three-year awareness campaign on the dangers of smoking and on healthy diet (ash.org.uk).

In February of 1988, the Health Education Authority (HEA) launched "Smoking and Me", which was aimed at educating 12 and 13 year olds on the dangers of smoking (ash.org.uk). By October of 1989, the European Council banned tobacco advertising across Europe, including the UK. In January of 1990, MPs, activist and members of the public, led by Esther Rantzen and Richard Branson, launched "Parents against Tobacco". Their aim was to pressure the government to put in place legislation to protect young children and the underaged Protection of Children (Tobacco) Act 1986.

In June of 1991, the government published a Green Paper, "The Health of the Nation", which proposed to reduce overall smoking by one-third by the year 2000 (Akehurst and Hutton 1991). That same month, the Children and Young Persons (Protection from Tobacco) Act 1991 was introduced. This increased the penalties for selling tobacco to those under 16 years of age. The following month, 29 organisations representing 85,000 doctors in the UK launched Doctors for Tobacco Law. This group organised a demonstration outside Rothmans International and this this was widely covered by the media. They linked the death of every smoker to the company's profit of up to £35,250.

In line with the European Commission requirement, the government also announced larger health warnings for tobacco packaging (Feldman and Bayer 2009). This was the first time that health warnings were brought under legal control rather than being covered by voluntary agreements. In response to this, the UK tobacco industry expressed concern about the new size of the health warnings and then sued the UK government (ash.org.uk). This act alone bought the tobacco industry time, but may also have been an exercise of economic power designed to cause delay in policy intervention. That same month, the HEA published "The Smoking Epidemic" and revealed that tobacco-related diseases in the UK claim 111,000 lives every year (ash.org.uk).

In July of 1992, the UK government published the White Paper "The Health of the Nation". This paper was criticised for outlawing tobacco advertising completely (DoH 1992). However, the paper offered to increase the target for public tobacco consumption. It also promised to introduce legislation to allow licensed taxi drivers to ban smoking in their vehicles (DoH 1992). In May of 1997, the Queen's speech included a bill to outlaw tobacco advertising (Queen's Speech 1997). Following the Queen's speech, Tessa Jowell, the UK Minister of State for Public Health, stated that

> The Government is fully committed to banning tobacco advertising. This is an essential first step in building an effective strategy to deal with smoking. (Jowell 1997)

In December of 1998, the Secretary of State for Health presented a White Paper on Tobacco by Command of Her Majesty. This made it the first tobacco bill published by the UK government. The bill acknowledges the role of the government in curbing the dangers of tobacco (The UK Government White Paper 1998).

References

(1997). On the opening of Parliament by her Majesty Queen Elizabeth II Queen of the United Kingdom.

Akehurst, R., & Hutton, J. (1991). *The health of the nation': An economic perspective on target setting*. York: Centre for Health Economics, University of York.

Alderson, M., Lee, P., & Wang, R. (1985). Risks of lung cancer, chronic bronchitis, ischaemic heart disease, and stroke in relation to type of cigarette smoked. *Journal of Epidemiology and Community Health, 39*, 286–293.

ash.org.uk. Key dates in the history of anti-tobacco campaigning. In A. O. S. A. Health (Ed.). http://ash.org.uk/information-and-resources/briefings/key-dates-in-the-history-of-anti-tobacco-campaigning/. Accessed 16 May 2016.

Auerbach, O., Forman, J. B., Gere, J. B., Kassouny, D. Y., Muehsam, G. E., Petrick, T. G., Smolin, H. J., & Stout, A. P. (1957). Changes in the bronchial epithelium in relation to smoking and cancer of the lung; a report of progress. *The New England Journal of Medicine, 256,* 97–104.

BBC. (2009). *Yet another BDO/PDC article* [Online]. Available: http://news.bbc.co.uk/dna/606/A50672289. Accessed 18 June 2014.

BBC news. (1956). *Minister rejects anti-smoking lobby.* http://news.bbc.co.uk/onthisday/hi/dates/stories/may/7/newsid_2518000/2518245.stm. Accessed 18 June 2015.

Bock, F. G., & Moore, G. E. (1959). Carcinogenic activity of cigarette-smoke condensate. I. Effect of trauma and remote x irradiation. *Journal of the National Cancer Institute, 22,* 401–411.

Chang, S. C. (1957). Microscopic properties of whole mounts and sections of human bronchial epithelium of smokers and nonsmokers. *Cancer, 10,* 1246–1262.

CHSC & SACCR. (1951). The central health services committee, Standing Advisory Committee on Cancer and Radiotherapy Note by the Secretary, 1951, 27 March [L&D Gov/Pro 4].

CHSC & SACCR. (1953). Central Health Services Committee, Standing Advisory Committee on Cancer and Radiotherapy. Note by the Secretary, 1953, February [L&D Gov/Pro 14].

CHSC & SACCR. (1956). Cancer and radiotherapy, smoking and cancer of the lung, Note by the Ministry of Health. In Central Health Services Committee, S. A. C. (ed.).

Clarke, R. W. S. (1962). Chairman of Imperial Tobacco, Statement to Shareholders.

DoH. (1992). *The health of the nation: A strategy for health in England.* London: HMSO.

Doll, R., & Hill, A. B. (1950). Smoking and carcinoma of the lung. *British Medical Journal, 2*(4682), 739.

Doll, R., & Hill, A. B. (1952). A study of the aetiology of carcinoma of the lung. *British Medical Journal, 2*(4797), 1271–1286.

Doll, R., & Hill, A. B. (1954). The mortality of doctors in relation to their smoking habits. *British Medical Journal, 1,* 1451.

Doll, R., & Hill, A. B. (1964). Mortality in relation to smoking: Ten years' observations of British doctors. *British Medical Journal, 1,* 1399.

Doll, R., Hill, A. B., & Kreyberg, L. (1957). The significance of cell type in relation to the aetiology of lung cancer. *British Journal of Cancer, 11,* 43.

Dorn, H. F. (1959). Tobacco consumption and mortality from cancer and other diseases. *Public Health Reports, 74,* 581.

Engelbreth-Holm, J., & Ahlmann, J. (1957). Production of carcinoma in ST/Eh mice with cigarette tar. *Acta pathologica et microbiologica Scandinavica, 41,* 267–272.

Eysenck, H., Tarrant, M., Woolf, M., & England, L. (1960). Smoking and personality. *British Medical Journal, 1,* 1456.
Feldman, E. A., & Bayer, R. (2009). *Unfiltered: Conflicts over tobacco policy and public health.* Cambridge, MA: Harvard University Press.
Fisher, R. A. (1958). Lung cancer and cigarettes? *Nature, 182,* 108.
Fisher, S. R. A. (1959). *Smoking: The cancer controversy: Some attempts to assess the evidence.* London: Oliver and Boyd.
Gellhorn, A. (1958). The cocarcinogenic activity of cigarette tobacco tar. *Cancer Research, 18,* 510–517.
Glantz, S. A., & Forbes, E. R. (1996). *The cigarette papers* (Vol. 17). Berkeley: University of California Press.
Haenszel, W., Shimkin, M. B., & Mantel, N. (1958). A retrospective study of lung cancer in women. *Journal of the National Cancer Institute, 21*(5), 825–842.
Hammond, E. C., & Horn, D. (1954). The relationship between human smoking habits and death rates: A follow-up study of 187.
Hilding, A. C. (1956). On cigarette smoking, bronchial carcinoma and ciliary action: Experimental study on the filtering action of cow's lungs, the deposition of tar in the bronchial tree and removal by ciliary action. *New England Journal of Medicine, 254,* 1155–1160.
Hughes, D. (2012). Archive: Smokers in 1962 react to the report. BBC News Health.
Jowell, T. (1997). The Tobacco Advertising and Promotion Bill [HL] Bill 112 of 2001-02. Cited in The Tobacco Advertising and Promotion Bill [HL] Bill 112 of 2001-02 (page 19). https://researchbriefings.files.parliament.uk/documents/RP02-20/RP02-20.pdf. Accessed 15 April 2016.
Kotin, P., Falk, H. L., & Thomas, M. I. (1956). *Production of skin tumors in mice with oxidation products of aliphatic hydrocarbons.* United States: N. p. https://doi.org/10.1002/1097-0142(195609/10)9:5<905::AID-CNCR2820090505>3.0.CO;2-Y. U.S. Department of Energy Office of Scientific and Technical Information.
Leuchtenberger, C., Leuchtenberger, R., Doolin, P. F., & Shaffer, P. (1958). A correlated histological, cytological, and cytochemical study of the tracheobronchial tree and lungs of mice exposed to cigarette smoke. I. Bronchitis with atypical epithelial changes in mice exposed to cigarette smoke. *Cancer, 11,* 490–506.
Levin, M. L., Goldstein, H., & Gerhardt, P. R. (1950). Cancer and tobacco smoking: A preliminary report. *Journal of the American Medical Association, 143,* 336–338.
Libal, Joyce. (2014). *Putting out the fire: Smoking and the law.* Broomall: Mason Crest Publishers. https://books.google.co.uk/books?redir_esc=y&id=BJUPBQAAQBAJ&q=unbalanced+picture#v=snippet&q=unbalanced%20picture&f=false

Lopez, A. D. (1999). Measuring the health hazards of tobacco: Commentary/AD Lopez.
Lyons, M. J., & Johnston, H. (1957). Chemical investigation of the neutral fraction of cigarette smoke tar. *British Journal of Cancer, 11*, 554.
McCormick, A. (1962). Smoking and Health: Policy on Research, Minutes of Southampton Meeting.
Orris, L., Van Duuren, B. L., Kosak, A. I., Nelson, N., & Schmitt, F. L. (1958). The carcinogenicity for mouse skin and the aromatic hydrocarbon content of cigarette-smoke condensates. *Journal of the National Cancer Institute, 21*(3), 557–561.
Partridge, E. J. (1956). 9 March, 1956. RE: Letter from representative of tobacco industry to Sir John Hawton. Type to Hawton, S. J.
Peto, R., Darby, S., Deo, H., Silcocks, P., Whitley, E., & Doll, R. (2000). Smoking, smoking cessation, and lung cancer in the UK since 1950: Combination of national statistics with two case-control studies. *British Medical Journal, 321*, 323–329.
Pollock, D. (1999). *Denial & delay: The political history of smoking and health, 1951–1964: Scientists, government and industry as seen in the papers at the Public Records Office*. London: Action on Smoking and Health.
Protection of Children (Tobacco) Act. (1986). Chapter 34. http://www.legislation.gov.uk/ukpga/1986/34/introduction
RCP. (1962). A report of the Royal College of Physicians on smoking in relation to cancer of the lung and other diseases. In Report, R. C. O. P. (Ed.). https://www.rcplondon.ac.uk/sites/default/files/smoking-and-health1962.pdf. Royal College of Physicians.
RCP. (1971). *Smoking or Health*. London: Pitman Medical Publishing Company, Royal College of Physicians.
RCP. (1992). Smoking and the young. In *Physicians*, R. C. O. (Ed.).
Report of Special Master. (1998). Findings of fact, conclusions of law and recommendations regarding non-liggett privilege claims, March.
Schwartz, D., & Denoix, P. F. (1957). L'enquête française sur l'étiologie du cancer broncho-pulmonaire. Rôle du tabac. *La Semaine des Hopitaux de Paris, 33*, 424–437.
Sheehy, P. (1980). P. Sheehy. Letter to the BBC.
Smith, A. (1982). Sponsorship of sport by tobacco companies. *British Medical Journal (Clinical Research Ed.), 284*, 660.
Stocks, P. (1958). *Cancer incidence in North Wales and Liverpool region in relation to habits and environment. IX. Smoke and smoking*. British Empire Cancer Campaign 35th Annual Report.
Taylor, P. (1984). *Quoted in smoke ring - The politics of tobacco*. London: Bodley Head.

Taylor, P. (1985). *The smoke ring: Tobacco, money and international politics*. London: Sphere.
Teague, C. (1953). Survey of cancer research with emphasis upon possible carcinogens from tobacco. RJR document dated February, 2.
The Guardian. (2010). *From the archive, 28 June 1957: One in eight of heavy smokers "doomed"*. https://www.theguardian.com/theguardian/2010/jun/28/archive-one-in-eight-of-heavy-smokers-doomed-1957. Accessed 15 June 2015.
The UK Government White Paper. (1998). Policy paper on a white paper on tobacco. https://www.gov.uk/government/publications/a-white-paper-on-tobacco. Accessed 14 Mar 2015.
Tobacco, C. O. I. 17 March, 1953. (1953). RE: The Chairman of Imperial Tobacco to Share holders. Type to SHAREHOLDERS.
Todd, G. F. (1962). Comments on the report on smoking and health by a committee of the Royal College of Physicians, 1962; Assessment of comments made by Mr. Todd of the TMSC for research into the effects of smoking on health on the report of the Royal College of Physicians.
Turner, A. D. C. (1987). Tobacco-sponsored sport on television. *The Lancet, 330*(8561), 747. https://doi.org/10.1016/S0140-6736(87)91111-1
Van Duuren, B. L. (1958). Identification of some polynuclear aromatic hydrocarbons in cigarette-smoke condensate. *Journal of the National Cancer Institute, 21,* 1–16.
WHO. (2016). *Tobacco explained: The truth about the tobacco industry …in its own words. Page 8, 14.* https://www.who.int/tobacco/media/en/Tobacco Explained.pdf. Accessed March 2016.
Wynder, E. L., & Graham, E. A. (1950). Tobacco smoking as a possible etiologic factor in bronchiogenic carcinoma: A study of six hundred and eighty-four proved cases. *Journal of the American Medical Association, 143*(4), 329–336.
Wynder, E. L., & Wright, G. (1957). A study of tobacco carcinogenesis. I. The primary fractions. *Cancer, 10,* 255–271.
Wynder, E. L., Graham, E. A., & Croninger, A. B. (1953). Experimental production of carcinoma with cigarette tar. *Cancer Research, 13*(12), 855–864.
Wynder, E. L., Wright, G., & Lam, J. (1958). A study of tobacco carcinogenesis. V. The role of pyrolysis. *Cancer, 11,* 1140–1148.

The UK MMR Vaccine Debate

THE MMR VACCINE DEBATE (1998 AND 2000)

The technical debate relating to the MMR vaccination in UK originated from research that was conducted at London's Royal Free Hospital and led by Dr. Andrew Wakefield. This study published in *The Lancet* in February of 1998 suggested that there was a potential link between the MMR vaccine and regressive behavioural disorders after describing 12 children aged between three and ten years (Wakefield et al. 1998). In the paper, Wakefield et al. (1998) suggested that there was a possible environmental trigger to the children's behaviour and explained that most of the parents (of 8 of the 12 children) noted a change in these behaviours following MMR vaccination (Wakefield et al. 1998). A press release by Royal Free Hospital on the eve of the publication stated that

> Researchers at the Royal Free Hospital School of Medicine may have discovered a new syndrome in children involving a new inflammatory bowel disease and autism ... The study identified a possible link between gut disorder in children and autism. In the majority of cases the onset of symptoms occurred after the MMR vaccination. We clearly need further research to examine this new syndrome, and to look into [any] possible relation to the MMR vaccine. (Royal Free Hospital Press Release 1992, cited in Deer 2010)

As a precautionary measure, Wakefield called for the suspension of the triple injection in favour of single vaccines until the combination MMR vaccine was ruled out as a possible environmental trigger. He said that

It's a moral issue for me. ... and I can't support the continued use of these three vaccines given in combination until this issue has been resolved. (Deer 2004)

A number of ethical and honesty issues surrounding the MMR study must be mentioned from the outset. First, Andrew Wakefield was accused of using children who were already showing signs of autism in order to prove his theory (Novella 2009). Some have even alleged that he collected blood samples unethically from children at a birthday party, paying them £5.00 as a reward (Boseley 2010), or even faked his data (Deer 2004). Brian Deer, an investigative journalist, found that Wakefield had taken a large consulting fee from a solicitor who was representing clients pointing the finger at the MMR vaccine as the potential cause of their children's behavioural changes and who intended to file a case against the vaccine manufacturers (Deer 2008). In fact, 11 of the 12 children in his 1998 *Lancet* publication were found to be part of the litigation. It was also discovered that he had logged a patent to produce a new vaccine against measles known as the Transfer Factor. Wakefield had initially claimed that this vaccine was safer (Novella 2009) and could be used to treat inflammatory bowel disease (Boseley 2010). Ten of the co-authors of the *Lancet* study withdrew their names from the publication. The paper was also retracted by the editors of *The Lancet* on the basis that the authors had not disclosed any conflict of interest (Horton 2004).

Andrew Wakefield's claims were met with fierce scrutiny following the *Lancet* study and was followed by a request from Sir Kenneth Calman, the Chief Medical Officer (CMO), and the Medical Research Council. Thirty-seven experts formed an ad hoc committee, combining current expertise including child psychiatry, epidemiology, immunology and virology (Edwards 2001), and convened to review Wakefield's evidence and claims. The expert committee reviewed the associations between the measles virus and the MMR vaccine, and between inflammatory bowel disease and autism (MRC 1998). At the end of this meeting, the expert committee reached a conclusion that the evidence was insufficient to suggest that there was a relationship between the MMR vaccine and autism and bowel disorders like Crohn's disease and ulcerative colitis (MRC 1998, p. 3, cited in Fitzpatrick 2004).

> No evidence was presented to suggest that MMR vaccination gives rise to autism ... The age at which MMR is usually given coincides with the age at

which autism is often recognised; this does not mean that one causes the other ... A better understanding is needed of the causes of ... autism. (Thrower 1997)

The conclusion was signed by the CMO Sir Kenneth Calman on 27 March and then sent in a letter to every doctor in the UK (Calman 1998). Sir Kenneth Calman stated,

I strongly advise parents to continue to have their children immunised with the MMR vaccine. (BBC 1998b)

However, the director of Justice, Awareness & Basic Support (JABS) group raised a concern that more time was needed to consider the issue (Casiday 2005). JABS is a group launched in 1994 for and by parents who believe their children were damaged following childhood vaccination. In May of 1998, a 14-year Finnish study on adverse effect of vaccines did not reveal any association between the MMR vaccine and autism. A study published in July 2000 examined a historical vaccination project report maintained by the national board of health investigation (Peltola et al. 1998). The researchers performed a study with two prospective cohorts, examining the histories of the vaccines and charting 1.8 million individuals registered in the MMR vaccination programme in 1982. This also involved 3 million doses of vaccine that had been administered. The study found that only 173 serious reactions had been recorded as possibly being caused by the vaccine and 31 gastrointestinal symptoms identified; none of the children had developed autism according to the study (Peltola et al. 1998). The findings from this study were of vital significance, considering its large scope. David Walker, of the department of public health medicine, Durham county health authority, described Wakefield's association between the vaccine and the diseases as

Anecdotal reporting of a biased sample and has no place in a peer-reviewed journal. (Walker 1998)

In June of 1998, significant reduction in MMR vaccine uptake was found in Wales according to the Public Health Laboratory Service. This was after a study by Thomas et al. (1998), who found that there was a general decline in the number of people opting for the MMR vaccine. This signalled a mistrust or suspicion in the MMR immunisation programme and of government reassurances that the vaccine was safe. Parents' suspicions about the MMR vaccine may also have been linked to other previous events or controversies. For example, the Department of Health (DoH) withdrew two brands of vaccines used in Britain out of the three used at the time. The withdrawal was due to the suggestion that the mumps component of the MMR vaccine caused mild transient meningitis (Sugiura and Yamada 1991). The two brands that were withdrawn were Immravax by Merieux UK and Pluserix, due to the fact that they contained a strain of a mumps virus linked to meningitis. The third brand, MMR-II, used a strain of virus that carried a lower risk (Dyer 1994). MMR-II is manufactured by Merck Sharp and Dohme, who in response to the growing anxiety said,

> more than 150 million doses of MMR-II have been administered, establishing an unsurpassed record of safety and effectiveness. (Dyer 1994)

There was also the anti-vaccination movement in the Britain in the 1800s that may have further entrenched parents' suspicion of the claim that there is no causal relationship linking MMR vaccination to autism (Blume 2006). This distrust or suspicion was accentuated by already existing negative public attitudes to government authorities, resulting from previous public controversies, such as the BSE epidemic. In the case of BSE, government experts reversed their reassurances with the original message that BSE was of no threat to humans (Caplan 2000; Bellaby 2003; Murphy-Lawless 2003), impacting on their credibility. In July 1998, the government attempted to provide reassurance by sending over 2 million leaflets, distributed through 9000 GP surgeries and 156 health promotion units (BBC 1998a). The leaflet, "MMR-The Facts", published a clear message that there was no sufficient evidence that linked MMR vaccines, bowel disease and autism. The leaflet, produced by the DoH and the Health Education Authority (HEA), further stated that children could die from the diseases if they failed to take the MMR vaccination (BBC 1998a). In the leaflet, the government argued that

> The risk from the three diseases [is] greater than the risk of developing autism, which has not been proven.

By October of 1998, a pharmacist in Croydon, Surrey, Andrew McCoig, was reported to be supplying parents who were opting for the single injections. McCoig believed that parents should be given alternative options and should be able to exercise a choice about their child's immunisation (BBC 1998b). In June of 1999, a Medicines Control Agency-funded study reviewed almost 500 cases of autism but was unable to establish a relationship between the MMR vaccine and autism.

In August of 1999, a study in the *BMJ* found that single mumps vaccine offers no protection to children (Schlegel et al. 1999). This brand was once used in the UK. The significance of this paper is that it went beyond only verifying Wakefield's argument, and also investigated his suggested alternative to the triple injection. By November of 1999, about eight families had lodged a High Court injunction against MMR vaccine manufacturers. These families were represented by solicitor Richard Barr. It was also revealed that 350 families received legal aid in support of similar cases (Buncombe 1998, cited in Casiday 2005).

In December of 1999, an outbreak of measles occurred in North Dublin, Ireland, and lasted until July of 2000 (McBrien et al. 2003). During the outbreak, 844 suspected cases were recorded. This number is significant compared with 152 notifications between 1995 and 1999. Two (2) children died, out of the hundred and one (101) children who were hospitalised (McBrien et al. 2003). By the end of 1999, no other scientific study or evidence was able to verify Dr. Wakefield's claims. In February of 2000, a study by Kaye et al. (2001) published in the *BMJ* found a continuous rise in autism despite the rate of MMR vaccine administration remaining static. According to the study, "the explanation for the marked increase in risk of the diagnosis of autism in the past decade remains uncertain".

That same month in another publication co-authored by two other researchers, Dr. Wakefield suggested that their study found "an endoscopically and histologically consistent pattern of ileo-colonic pathology" in "a cohort of children with developmental disorders" (Wakefield et al. 2000, p. 2294). The study reviewed 60 cases of 'autistic enterocolitis' including 12 of the cases in the 1998 *Lancet* publication. The authors describe a "new variant" of inflammatory bowel disease that implicated the MMR vaccine (Wakefield et al. 2000).

The MRC commissioned another expert subgroup in April of 2000 to examine new evidence on inflammatory bowel disease and autism, and to examine evidence from the expert team of the Royal Free Hospital (Wakefield et al. 2000). The MRC criticised the study for cherry-picking evidence, describing it as a "self-selected group of patients" and adding that "the histological finding of ileal lymphoid-nodular hyperplasia may have been secondary to severe constipation" (MRC 2000, p. 4, cited in

Fitzpatrick 2004). The expert committee following their review reached the conclusion that "the case for 'autistic enterocolitis' had not been proven" (MRC 2000, p. 4, cited in Fitzpatrick 2004), calling for more research on inflammatory bowel disease (Fitzpatrick 2004).

In October of 2000, the Joint Committee on Vaccination and Immunisation (JCVI), Medicines Control Agency and the DoH reviewed a paper (supplied by the authors, Wakefield and Montgomery) that was due to be published by the end of the year. They all came to the conclusion that the yet unpublished paper provided no new or additional evidence to change its current view on MMR vaccination (Medicines Control Agency and Department of Health 2001). The study due to be published suggested that the MMR vaccine did not undergo a safety test. The Medicines Control Agency (MCA) and DoH accused the report of cherry-picking evidence, arguing that the triple MMR vaccine was safer for young children when compared to the single dose (which would be administered at a slow pace and increase the chances of parents missing one element of it).

THE MMR VACCINE DEBATE (2001–2003)

At the start of 2001, the UK government launched a £3 million in pounds awareness creation campaign to address the growing public concern about the MMR vaccine (Boseley 2001). The campaign was directed at parents and health professionals, a move which was criticised by the National Autistic Society, who stated that the government focus should be on research rather than advertising (Boseley 2001). Also in January, Wakefield revealed to the *Daily Telegraph* that he had evidence of 170 new cases of 'autistic syndrome'. According to him, health authorities had failed to adequately address the safety of the MMR vaccine (Fraser 2001b). *The Daily Mail* and other news media launched campaigns to back Dr. Wakefield (Deer 2011), who was at this point viewed as a genuine expert standing alone against powerful corporations and the government. At this time, newspaper reports revealed that 500 parents planned to sue the DoH, claiming that their children were damaged by vaccines. About 850 families received legal aid for this purpose (Hall 2001).

In June of 2001, further studies such as that by Farrington et al. (2001) proved that there was no relationship between the MMR vaccine and autism. The study re-analysed the data from the previous study commissioned by the MRC (Taylor et al. 1999) and reached a conclusion that the results did not show a link between the MMR vaccine and autism. Nevertheless, that same month, the Lothian division of the BMA requested that the BMA back single vaccines as an alternative for parents who refuse the MMR vaccine. In December of 2001, Dr. Wakefield resigned from the Royal Free Hospital, stating that

> I have been asked to go because my research results are unpopular ... I did not wish to leave but I have agreed to stand down in the hope that my going will take the political pressure off my colleagues and allow them to get on with the job of looking after the many sick children we have seen ... They have not sacked me. They cannot; I have not done anything wrong. I have no intention of stopping my investigations. (Fraser 2001a)

Also in December, the MRC published a report that found that the number of autistic cases had increased to 6 in 1000 children (MRC 2001). However, this increase was attributed to other factors including changes in how autism is defined. The report found no evidence that linked the MMR vaccine and autism and pointed to other environmental factors and genetics.

There were other key events that led to the social amplification of the risk associated with MMR vaccine. These included the Tony Blair and Neo Leo Saga, other scientific reports; Brian Deer's investigation and the General Medical Council (GMC) professional misconduct investigation. Some of these are discussed here.

Tony Blair and Neo Leo Saga

The government decision not to offer a single vaccination programme put the then prime minister, Tony Blair, in the spotlight. In December of 2001, MP Julie Kirkbride, the mother of a 14-month-old boy, asked Mr. Blair during Prime Minister's Questions if Blair's son Leo had received the MMR vaccine. Mr. Blair declined to answer, insisting on family privacy on medical matters. The prime minister's insistence on not saying whether Leo was given the triple injection further heightened suspicion about the vaccine's safety. This seemly trivial event became the centre of attention in 2001, with 32% of media featuring this story (Speers and Lewis 2004). The Tony Blair saga was brought to an end in February 2002, when *The Independent* revealed that Leo Blair had been given the MMR vaccine

(Dillon 2002). However, the prime minister declined to confirm this based on privacy grounds. Other factors were also blamed for amplifying the risk of the MMR vaccine. Wakefield, for instance, blamed the MMR crisis on the removal of choice by the government, stating that

> What precipitated this [MMR] crisis was the removal of the single vaccine, the removal of choice, and that is what has caused the furore—because the doctors, the gurus, are treating the public as though they are some kind of moronic mass who cannot make an informed decision for themselves. (Wakefield 2002)

Parents were to give voluntarily consent for their children to be vaccinated. However, one parent, frustrated about the fact that she was not given an option, said,

> We were angry that we were not given a choice, that it had to be the combined three together, why they couldn't split it … We were told no you couldn't … we were never given that choice, we were just told this is how it is … why are we not allowed to have it, why is there not the option to have any of those three separate vaccines? (Evans et al. 2001)

In February of 2002, the government launched its own campaign including television appeals by the CMO and open letters to GP surgeries. The aim was to reassure parents, presenting them with information so they could make informed decisions. The politics of the MMR debate nevertheless continued to be important. In June, the then Mayor of London, Ken Livingstone, announced that he would choose to use the single vaccines for his child who was at the time still unborn (BBC 2002). In a statement to BBC Radio Five Live, he said he would be giving his child separate injections, when the time came, to guard against mumps, measles and rubella. However, the chairman of the BMA, Dr. Ian Bogle, criticised him, urging him to apologise and retract the statement. In October of 2002, the legal aid for more than 1000 parents accusing MMR vaccine manufacturers of damaging their children was stopped (Martin 2003).

As the debate progressed, the government realised it needed to do more than reassure parents and also had to provide information about what is known scientifically to both health practitioners and the public. The initial government reassuring response and one-way risk communication model was seen to be ineffective, since MMR uptake was for the first time on the decline in some parts of the country. Perhaps, where effective feedback processes were initiated, the outcome may have been different. This raises questions about whether the media scare alone can be held responsible for the decline in MMR vaccine uptake, or whether the one-way and ineffective risk communication approach of policymakers and health practitioners, who were keen to offer reassurances to concerned parents, are also significant. Other factors that may also have partly influenced the debate were the fact that the MMR vaccine debate came after the BSE inquiry, which occupied the attention of two CMOs in England and Wales, and occurred at the start of the Labour Government. These are all possible factors that could have influenced and shaped the social amplification (or attenuation) of the MMR vaccine debate.

The analysis of the MMR vaccine debate carried out through the PERC framework is presented in Chap. 7. However, the conclusion that can be drawn from the analysis of the evolving events carried out in this chapter is that there is a strong relationship between over-use of power of experts by stakeholder groups and social amplification (or attenuation) of risk. This is evidenced by Wakefield's research (that is marred by unethical behaviour) and his incorrect suggestion that the MMR vaccine is linked to autism despite the fact that his study did not constitute proof. When this is combined with vested interests (such as those seen in the case of Wakefield), this could present a dangerous and salient avenue of power in public health risk communication that may go unnoticed or unscrutinised because of perceived credibility of technical expertise that may allow social amplification (or attenuation) of risk to thrive.

REFERENCES

BBC. (1998a, September 4). Health MMR leaflets seek to reassure parents. *BBC News*.
BBC. (1998b). Sci/Tech: 'No link' between vaccine and autism. *BBC News*.
BBC. (2002, July 3). London Mayor warned over MMR defiance. *Mail Online*.
Bellaby, P. (2003). Communication and miscommunication of risk: Understanding UK parents' attitudes to combined MMR vaccination. *BMJ, 327*, 725.
Blume, S. (2006). Anti-vaccination movements and their interpretations. *Social Science & Medicine, 62*, 628–642.
Boseley, S. (2001). Doctor's green light for MMR campaign. *The Guardian*. https://www.theguardian.com/society/2001/nov/20/publichealth. Accessed 18 Jan 2016.

Boseley, S. (2010). *Andrew Wakefield case highlights the importance of ethics in science* [Online]. Available: https://www.theguardian.com/society/2010/may/24/andrew-wakefield-analysis-ethics-science. Accessed 17 Jan 2017.

Buncombe, A. (1998). Measles jab withdrawn due to 'high demand'. *The Independent*, p. 5. London.

Calman, K. (1998). Measles, mumps and rubella, vaccine and Chron's disease and autism. Dear doctor letter from the chief medical officer. March 1998 PL/CMO/98/2.

Caplan, P. (2000). Eating British beef with confidence: A consideration of consumers' responses to BSE in Britain. In *Risk revisited* (pp. 184–203). London: Pluto Press.

Casiday, R. E. (2005). *Risk conceptualisations, trust and decision-making in the face of contradictory information: The case of MMR*. Durham: Durham University.

Deer, B. (2004). MMR: The truth behind the crisis. *Sunday Times*.

Deer, B. (2010). Wakefield's "autistic enterocolitis" under the microscope. *BMJ, 340*, c1127.

Deer, B. (2011). How the case against the MMR vaccine was fixed. *BMJ, 342*, c5347.

Dillon, J. (2002). Focus: Child health – MMR. An end to the did-they, didn't-they saga of little Leo's jab; The Blairs' secret is out-their youngest son has had the controversial vaccine. But who told the press? *The Independent*.

DoH, M. A. (2001). Combined measles, mumps and rubella vaccines: Response of the Medicines Control Agency and Department of Health to issues raised in papers published in *Adverse drug reactions and toxicological reviews*.

Dyer, C. (1994). Families win support for vaccine compensation claim. *BMJ, 309*, 759.

Edwards, C. (2001). Is the MMR vaccine safe? *Western Journal of Medicine, 174*, 197.

Evans, M., Stoddart, H., Condon, L., Freeman, R., Grizzell, M., & Mullen, R. (2001). Parents' perspectives on the MMR immunisation: A focus group study. *British Journal of General Practice, 51*, 904–910.

Farrington, C., Miller, E., & Taylor, B. (2001). MMR and autism: Further evidence against a causal association. *Vaccine, 19*, 3632–3635.

Fitzpatrick, M. (2004). *MMR and autism: What parents need to know*. London: Routledge.

Fraser, L. (2001a, December 2). Anti-MMR doctor is forced out. *The Telegraph*.

Fraser, L. (2001b, January 21). MMR doctor links 170 cases of autism to vaccine. *The Telegraph Newspaper*.

Hall, C. (2001, January 26). Mother of five children with autism to sue over MMR jabs. *The Telegraph*.

Horton, R. (2004). A statement by the editors of The Lancet. *The Lancet, 363*, 820–821.

Kaye, J. A., del Mar Melero-Montes, M., & Jick, H. (2001). Mumps, measles, and rubella vaccine and the incidence of autism recorded by general practitioners: A time trend analysis. *BMJ, 322*, 460–463.

Martin, N. (2003). Parents seeking MMR compensation lose legal aid for court fight. *The Telegraph*.

McBrien, J., Murphy, J., Gill, D., Cronin, M., O'Donovan, C., & Cafferkey, M. T. (2003). Measles outbreak in Dublin, 2000. *The Pediatric Infectious Disease Journal, 22*, 580–584.

MRC. (2001). MRC review of autism research. In M. R. C. Report (Ed.), *The Medical Research Council*. http://www.mrc.ac.uk/news/publications/autism-research-review/

Murphy-Lawless, J. (2003). Risk, ethics, and the public space: The impact of BSE and foot-and-mouth disease on public thinking. In B. H. Harthorn & L. Oaks (Eds.), *Risk, culture, and health inequality: Shifting perceptions of danger and blame* (pp. 209–230). Westport: Praeger.

Novella, S. (2009). Autism-vaccine link researcher Andrew Wakefield accused of faking his data. *Skeptical Inquirer*.

Peltola, H., Patja, A., Leinikki, P., Valle, M., Davidkin, I., & Paunio, M. (1998). No evidence for measles, mumps, and rubella vaccine-associated inflammatory bowel disease or autism in a 14-year prospective study. *The Lancet, 351*, 1327–1328.

Schlegel, M., Osterwalder, J. J., Galeazzi, R. L., & Vernazza, P. L. (1999). Comparative efficacy of three mumps vaccines during disease outbreak in Eastern Switzerland: Cohort study. *BMJ, 319*, 352.

Speers, T., & Lewis, J. (2004). Journalists and jabs: Media coverage of the MMR vaccine. *Communication & Medicine, 1*, 171–181.

Sugiura, A., & Yamada, A. (1991). Aseptic meningitis as a complication of mumps vaccination. *The Pediatric Infectious Disease Journal, 10*, 209–213.

Taylor, B., Miller, E., Farrington, C., Petropoulos, M.-C., Favot-Mayaud, I., Li, J., & Waight, P. A. (1999). Autism and measles, mumps, and rubella vaccine: No epidemiological evidence for a causal association. *The Lancet, 353*, 2026–2029.

Thomas, D. R., Salmon, R., & King, J. (1998). Rates of first measles-mumps-rubella immunisation in Wales (UK). *The Lancet, 351*, 1927.

Thrower. (1997). Memorandum by Mr David Thrower. Item 323. https://publications.parliament.uk/pa/cm199899/cmselect/cmhealth/549/99072716.htm. Accessed 16 Mar 2016.

Walker, D. R. (1998). Autism, inflammatory bowel disease, and MMR vaccine. *The Lancet, 351*(9112), 1355. https://doi.org/10.1016/S0140-6736(98)26018-1

Wakefield, A. J. (2002). Why I owe it to parents to question triple vaccine. *Sunday Herald*. Archived from the original on 3 August 2003.

Wakefield, A. J., Murch, S. H., Anthony, A., Linnell, J., Casson, D., Malik, M., Berelowitz, M., Dhillon, A. P., Thomson, M. A., & Harvey, P. (1998). RETRACTED: Ileal-lymphoid-nodular hyperplasia, non-specific colitis, and pervasive developmental disorder in children. *The Lancet, 351*, 637–641.

Wakefield, A., Anthony, A., Murch, S., Thomson, M., Montgomery, S. M., Davies, S., O'Leary, J., Berelowitz, M., & Walker-Smith, J. A. (2000). Enterocolitis in children with developmental disorders. *The American Journal of Gastroenterology, 95*, 2285–2295.

CHAPTER 6

The Sugar Debate

THE EVOLUTION OF THE UK SUGAR DEBATE

The emergence of the sugar debate in the UK dates back to the book titled *Pure, White and Deadly* by John Yudkin in 1978 that associates sugar intake with several health conditions and heart diseases (Yudkin 1988). However, the comparative analysis carried out in this study linking sugar intake and other diseases amongst different populations was considered weak and inadequate evidence on which to base any valuable conclusions. This, combined with powerful economic interests around sugar as a commercial product, meant that the association between sugar and poor health remained a contentious issue over many decades to come.

THE SUGAR PROBLEM

The core concern relating to sugar as a public health issue related to the assumption that high consumption of sugar from food or drinks leads to weight gain and obesity. This then has a knock-on effect on health, bringing about conditions such as heart disease, type 2 diabetes and tooth decay (Ludwig et al. 2001; Apovian 2004). Concerns around sugar consumption were further fuelled by recent studies conducted in England. For example, one of the studies found that around one in four adults in England was considered obese and another 37% considered overweight (Tedstone et al. 2015). In the report, one in ten year olds, and 19% of those in the age bracket of 10 to 11 years, were obese. Similarly, 34% and 46% of 12 and 15 year olds were found to have tooth decay in 2013 (Tedstone et al. 2015). More worrying is the suggestion that children from the poorest communities are twice as likely to be overweight and obese when compared with children from wealthy communities for same age groups (Tedstone et al. 2015).

Aside from these health consequences, sugar-related conditions such as the rise of obesity is increasingly being seen as one of the biggest challenges to the National Health Service (NHS), especially in terms of cost. For example, the cost of obesity to the NHS was put at £5.1bn per year (Campbell 2015b). The Chief Executive of NHS England, Simon Stevens, likened this to "the new smoking" challenge (Campbell 2015a). Similarly, the WHO describes the sugar problem especially in young children as "one of the most serious public health challenges for the 21st Century" (WHO 2019).

Events Prior to 2015

In 2003, the WHO put out a recommendation that "free sugars" should be less than 10% of our diet (WHO 2003). They describe free sugars as "sugars added to the food by the manufacturer, cook or consumer, plus sugars naturally present in honey, syrups and fruit juices" (WHO 2014). This follows a review of scientific evidence by 30 independent experts who concluded that sugar should be set to an average of 10%, a target in line with another 23 national reports and recommendations (Boseley 2003).

The WHO can be seen to shape research around the sugar debate on the international level, and scientific expertise is called upon to help make sense of the sugar problem and was thus influential in the early stages of the sugar debate. This recommendation by the WHO put the burden of proof on the shoulders of the sugar industry, who had to prove that any limit above 10% was safe for consumption. Within the UK, this burden of proof was also shared by the UK public health institution, who are responsible for public health and safety. Other stakeholders within the sugar debate are pressure groups, the medical profession, the sugar industry, media and the UK government.

The response of the sugar industry in the aftermath of the WHO 2003 recommendation reflects the contentions that existed within and between the scientific community on the one hand and industry on the other. For example, the US sugar industry, following the WHO 2003 recommendation, fiercely challenged the WHO's 10% recommendation, calling on the organisation to scrap the guideline. Their challenge was written in a letter sent to Gro Harlem Brundtland, the Director General of the WHO, by associates of the sugar industry (Sugar Association Letter to WHO 2003). In the letter, the industry expressed their displeasure, stating that they were determined to "exercise every avenue available to expose the dubious nature" of the WHO's diet and nutrition report (Guardian 2003). The main issue of contention was around the 10% limit put on dietary sugar consumption. The industry claimed that another report from the Institute of Medicine put the safe limit of sugar intake in food and drink at 25% (Sugar Association Letter to WHO 2003). However, the Institute of Medicine was quick to warn that their report made no such recommendations (Boseley 2003). The sugar industry went further, to challenge the £260 m public funding to the WHO, stating that

> Taxpayers' dollars should not be used to support misguided, non-science-based reports which do not add to the health and well-being of Americans, much less the rest of the world, ... If necessary we will promote and encourage new laws which require future WHO funding to be provided only if the organisation accepts that all reports must be supported by the preponderance of science. (Boseley 2003)

These unfolding events highlight that the initial response of the sugar industry was to attack any scientific evidence made against sugar and to discredit the intentions of any organisation associated with it.

Science, Evidence and Power Strategy

In 2013, the WHO, determined to update their recommendation, commissioned a report to review scientific evidence on the effect of increasing and decreasing sugar consumption on body weight in both adults and children. The report, published in the *BMJ* (Te Morenga et al. 2013) is significant as it gathered scientific evidence from over 68 existing studies (30 of which were randomised controlled trials and the remaining 38 were cohort studies) (Te Morenga et al. 2013). The study found that higher sugar intake resulted in increase in body weight. In another comprehensive study carried out by Moynihan and Kelly (2014), significant detrimental impact of sugar was found on dental caries, and this progresses with age and can be lifelong. Following these studies, the WHO said:

The evidence shows, first, that adults who consume less sugars have lower body weight and, second, that increasing the amount of sugars in the diet is associated with a weight increase. In addition, research shows that children with the highest intakes of sugar-sweetened drinks are more likely to be overweight or obese than children with a low intake of sugar-sweetened drinks. The recommendation is further supported by evidence showing higher rates of dental caries (commonly referred to as tooth decay) when the intake of free sugars is above 10% of total energy intake compared with an intake of free sugars below 10% of total energy intake. (WHO 2015)

Following this evidence, the WHO set out two *strong* and *conditional* recommendations. There was a strong recommendation to reduce intake of sugar to less than 10% of dietary intake. The conditional recommendation was for less than 5% of total sugar in the diet.

Following this, WHO opened a public consultation to gather public views on its recommendations in March of 2014. However, some would argue that the public should have been engaged with earlier on, for example, in the framing and shaping of the research agenda that informed the sugar research and then debate. This consultation attracted 170 comments from international and government agencies, industries, NGOs, academic institutions and individuals. The WHO further gathered expert opinion in a review process that took place in 2014; outcomes from both events were reflected in the final guideline (WHO 2015). This again highlights the role of technical expertise in shaping public debate about risk as this evolves.

Within the literature, the sugar industry attack on science and the bid to control research and evidence was well documented in three studies: Bes-Rastrollo et al. (2013), Goldman (2014) and Kearns et al. (2015). These studies revealed how the sugar industry tried to influence science and research, and through this to delay or prevent policy interventions that could be detrimental to the industry. For example, Bes-Rastrollo et al. (2013) concluded that studies that indicated that they had conflict of interest were up to 5 times more likely to discredit the relationship between sugar and weight gain. Goldman (2014) identified several ways in which the industry attempted to influence the sugar debate and these include undermining scientific evidence, publicising false information through multiple and supposedly credible outlets, engaging scientific expertise and using scientific language to shape the debate, and engaging policymakers by establishing stakeholder relationships. Similarly, Kearns et al. (2015) identified several tactics used by the industry to influence the sugar debate and policy regulation. These include funding research collaborations and aligning research agendas with key players, and establishing relationships with institutional expert groups.

Subsequently, the UK medical community encouraged the UK government to adopt WHO recommendations. In July of 2015, the UK Scientific Advisory Committee on Nutrition (SACN) published a report titled "Carbohydrates and Health". The report, similar to the WHO, also made the recommendation that sugar intake from the age of two should not exceed 5% of total dietary energy (SACN 2015). The report also recommended that fibre should account for 50% of our diet. This recommendation is significant as it was the first move from the SACN to recommend reduction in any specific food intake.

The Sugar Tax Argument

In July of 2015, the BMA advised the UK government to introduce a 20% tax on sugar to fight the challenge of obesity and type 2 diabetes. This argument was further strengthened with subsequent studies continuing to implicate sugar. For example, a University of Cambridge study links 8000 cases of type 2 diabetes to sugar consumption (Imamura et al. 2015). In response to the call for a tax on sugar, Gavin Partington, of the British Soft Drinks Association, said,

> There is no evidence worldwide that taxes of this sort reduce obesity, and it is ironic that soft drinks are being singled out for tax when we've led the way in reducing sugar intake, down over 17% since 2012… We're also the only category to have set a 20% calorie reduction target for 2020. (Boseley 2016b)

In November of 2015, the International Diabetes Federation (IDF) also called on national government to use sugar taxes as a means of fighting obesity and type 2 diabetes (Hirschler 2016). In August of 2015, *Sugar Rush*, a documentary by Jamie Oliver, revealed evidence to show the scale of the sugar problem in the UK. In the documentary, one doctor reports on how some children needed to have all their teeth removed due to dental problems, pointing to sugary drinks as the key problem. At this point, the UK government continued to insist that no sugar tax would be imposed on sugary products. The then prime minister, David Cameron, said that there were "more effective ways of tackling obesity" (Dathan and Cooper 2015).

In October of 2015, *Public Health England* (*PHE*) published a report titled *The Evidence for Action* (Tedstone et al. 2015). This sugar report recommends the introduction of a 10–20% tax on high-sugar products, stricter marketing regulation on unhealthy children's products and to develop innovative ways of reformulating products to have less sugar (Tedstone et al. 2015). This report called on ministers to take decisive steps to curb the growing challenge of obesity and health based on the convincing evidence that sugar was linked to increased body weight. This report, which drew a lot of attention within both the academic and public domains, can be seen to shape future control measures put in place to reduce public consumption of sugar.

There are several arguments both for and against a sugar tax (Niederdeppe et al. 2013). Arguments for a sugar tax have tended to highlight the potential health and financial benefits of a tax to other sectors of the economy. For example, a sugar tax could reduce health problems such as diabetes and obesity and this could have a positive impact by reducing the cost to the NHS (Mytton et al. 2012). Where an individual experience poor health, this is argued to bring about absenteeism, and lower productivity, and this could potentially increase the social cost associated with sugar consumption than any benefit to individual person or groups (Pettinger 2017). It is also estimated that a 20% sugar tax could raise billions in pounds for the government and this could be channelled positively to promote health care and healthy eating campaigns (BBC 2018). In addition, it is believed that a sugar tax would encourage organisations to come up with more innovative products that are healthier (Pettinger 2017).

On the other side of the debate, critics argue that a sugar tax could reduce the market share and profit from sugary products in a way that could impact on jobs due to increased cost to businesses (Rodionova 2016). There is also the argument that a sugar tax could encourage uptake of alcoholic drinks, while shifting consumer demands away from sugary drinks. There is also the nanny state argument: some argue that it is inappropriate to have the government deciding what the public should consume or how they should live their lives (Pettinger 2017).

Other national policy contexts were also relevant here (see, e.g., International Diabetes Federation Europe 2016). Several nations at this time had implemented a sugar tax, including Finland where a sugar tax has been in place since the 1940s, increasing taxes from 0.045€ per litre to 0.075€ in 2011. Can and ice cream taxes were also introduced in

2011. Similarly, Norway introduced a tax of 7.05 kroner, equivalent to 0.75€ per kilo, on refined sugar products and sugary drinks. In Hungary, a sugar tax was introduced on a number of products such as sugary drinks and prepackaged products in 2011. In 2012, France introduced a tax on sugary drinks of 0.075€ per litre. This shows the importance of the broader environmental context in shaping the debates that are brought to bear on risk.

UK Sugar Policy Decision (2016)

The year 2016 saw further pressure being put on the UK government. For example, a study by Queen Mary University experts in London concluded that a 40% reduction of sugary drinks could potentially prevent about 300,000 cases of type 2 diabetes within a five-year period. A total of 1.5 m cases of obesity could also be prevented within the same period. The government was then seen to delay its child obesity strategy publication. The strategy was due to be published in December but was delayed to January and then to February. However, it was not actually published until summer of 2016 (Boseley 2016a). The delay in the publication of this strategy in the UK was met with a great deal of anxiety and criticism amongst health campaigners. For example, Shirley Cramer, the Chief Executive of the Royal Society for Public Health, stated,

> Childhood obesity is a time bomb on which the clock is ticking, set to wreck the future health of our children and the sustainability of our NHS. There can be no excuse for delay or prevarication when we know – and the government knows – what must be done, especially if those delays are for political reasons. (Boseley 2016a)

Similarly, Professor Russell Viner, Royal College of Pediatrics and Child Health, expressed is frustration, saying that

> With every day that passes, more children are at risk of developing serious conditions associated with obesity. These include type 2 diabetes, high blood pressure and asthma. So yet another delay in the publication of the government's childhood obesity strategy gives great cause for concern. (Boseley 2016a)

In a surprising move in March of 2016, the UK government announced that it would introduce a UK-wide tax on sugary drinks or sugar-sweetened beverages in its annual provisions. Mr. Osborne, speaking to the House of Commons, says

> I am not prepared to look back at my time here in this Parliament, doing this job and say to my children's generation 'I'm sorry. We knew there was a problem with sugary drinks. We knew it caused disease. But we ducked the difficult decisions and we did nothing'. (Stewart 2016)

The government spokesperson suggested that the government wanted to encourage producer-led behavioural changes through reformulation and replacement of product portfolios with less sugary products.

A Change of Power Strategy by the Sugar Industry

Following the government announcement to introduce a sugar tax in its annual budget and with established evidence linking sugar and weight gain, the sugar industry can be seen to change its power strategy from one of attacking or attenuating the technical case made against sugar and its products to intensifying its lobbying of the government to influence its policy approach. For example, the sugar industry sponsored a drinks party at the Conservative Party conference, and according to a British Soft Drinks Association spokesperson:

> Anybody who believes this will have a marked effect on obesity needs to challenge that perception … We in the soft drinks industry are ahead of the game so it seems slightly odd we were the only product category singled out for the tax…. I'd like to welcome the business secretary here this evening and wish him well in his role. We want to work with government to help tackle obesity, but we believe that can be done without detriment to our industry or others, or the many small businesses we support. Thank you for listening. Please enjoy your wine. (Mason 2016)

The year 2016 also witnessed a change of government following the UK Leave vote in the 2016 European Union referendum. There were groups that were concerned about the potential for the sugar industry to take advantage of the change in government to water down any policy interventions considering that a sugar tax was proposed by the previous government (Mason 2016). Following a nine-week public consultation in the summer of 2016, a legislation on sugar levy was accepted by Parliament under the Finance Act 2017 (HM Revenue & Customs 2017). This levy came into effect in April 2018.

REFERENCES

Apovian, C. M. (2004). Sugar-sweetened soft drinks, obesity, and type 2 diabetes. *JAMA, 292*, 978–979.
BBC. (2018). *Sugar tax on soft drinks raises £154m* [Online]. Available: https://www.bbc.co.uk/news/business-46279224. Accessed 2 Jan 2019.
Bes-Rastrollo, M., Schulze, M. B., Ruiz-Canela, M., & Martinez-Gonzalez, M. A. (2013). Financial conflicts of interest and reporting bias regarding the association between sugar-sweetened beverages and weight gain: A systematic review of systematic reviews. *PLoS Medicine, 10*, E1001578.
Boseley, S. (2003). *Sugar industry threatens to scupper WHO* [Online]. Available: https://www.theguardian.com/society/2003/apr/21/usnews.food. Accessed 2 Feb 2019.
Boseley, S. (2016a). Childhood obesity strategy delayed further, government admits. *The Guardian.* https://www.theguardian.com/society/2016/feb/26/childhood-obesity-strategy-delayed-sugar-tax-unlikely. Accessed 3 Jan 2019.
Boseley, S. (2016b). *Price of sugary soft drinks could rise by 8p a can when tax introduced* [Online]. Available: https://www.theguardian.com/lifeandstyle/2016/dec/05/price-of-sugary-soft-drinks-could-rise-by-8p-a-can-when-tax-introduced. Accessed 2 Feb 2019.
Campbell, D. (2015a, July 13). Government delays publication of plans for reduction in UK's sugar intake. *The Guardian.*
Campbell, D. (2015b, October 23). Sugar and Britain's obesity crisis: The key questions answered. *The Guardian.*
Customs, H. R. (2017). *Draft legislation: Soft Drinks Industry Levy* [Online]. Available: https://www.gov.uk/government/consultations/draft-legislation-soft-drinks-industry-levy. Accessed 7 Feb 2017.
Dathan, M., & Cooper, C. (2015). *Sugar tax ruled out by David Cameron: 'There are more effective ways of tackling obesity'* [Online]. Available: https://www.independent.co.uk/news/uk/politics/david-cameron-rules-out-sugar-tax-there-are-more-effective-ways-of-tackling-obesity-a6704316.html. Accessed 2 Feb 2019.
Europe, I. D. F. (2016). *IDF Europe position on added sugar* [Online]. Available: http://www.eu-patient.eu/globalassets/library/publications/added-sugar-final_idf-europe-position.pdf. Accessed 20 Feb 2019.
Goldman, G. (2014). *Added sugar, subtracted science: How industry obscures science and undermines public health policy on sugar.* Cambridge, MA: Union of Concerned Scientists.

Guardian. (2003). *Sugar giants threaten WHO's funding* [Online]. Available: https://www.smh.com.au/world/sugar-giants-threaten-whos-funding-20030422-gdgn2k.html. Accessed 2 Feb 2018.

Hirschler, B. (2016). Diabetes experts tell G20 to tax sugar to save lives and money. *Reuters.*

Imamura, F., O'Connor, L., Ye, Z., Mursu, J., Hayashino, Y., Bhupathiraju, S. N., & Forouhi, N. G. (2015). Consumption of sugar sweetened beverages, artificially sweetened beverages, and fruit juice and incidence of type 2 diabetes: Systematic review, meta-analysis, and estimation of population attributable fraction. *BMJ, 351,* H3576.

Kearns, C. E., Glantz, S. A., & Schmidt, L. A. (2015). Sugar industry influence on the scientific agenda of the National Institute of Dental Research's 1971 National Caries Program: A historical analysis of internal documents. *PLoS Medicine, 12,* E1001798.

Ludwig, D. S., Peterson, K. E., & Gortmaker, S. L. (2001). Relation between consumption of sugar-sweetened drinks and childhood obesity: A prospective, observational analysis. *The Lancet, 357,* 505–508.

Mason, R. (2016). *Soft drinks industry lobbies government to dilute sugar tax* [Online]. Available: https://www.theguardian.com/lifeandstyle/2016/oct/21/soft-drinks-industry-lobbies-government-dilute-scrap-sugar-tax. Accessed 20 Feb 2019.

Moynihan, P., & Kelly, S. (2014). Effect on caries of restricting sugars intake: Systematic review to inform WHO guidelines. *Journal of Dental Research, 93,* 8–18.

Mytton, O. T., Clarke, D., & Rayner, M. (2012). Taxing unhealthy food and drinks to improve health. *BMJ, 344,* E2931.

Niederdeppe, J., Gollust, S. E., Jarlenski, M. P., Nathanson, A. M., & Barry, C. L. (2013). News coverage of sugar-sweetened beverage taxes: Pro-and antitax arguments in public discourse. *American Journal of Public Health, 103,* E92–E98.

Pettinger, T. (2017). *Sugar tax debate* [Online]. Economics. Available: https://www.economicshelp.org/blog/14884/economics/sugar-tax-debate/. Accessed 10 Jan 2019.

Rodionova, Z. (2016). *Sugar tax: UK businesses claim levy will result in job losses and higher prices* [Online]. Available: https://www.independent.co.uk/news/business/news/sugar-tax-uk-effects-obesity-levy-higher-prices-job-losses-businesses-claim-a7193351.html. Accessed 15 Jan 2019.

SACN. (2015). SACN carbohydrates and health report. In P. Health (Ed.), *The Scientific Advisory Committee on Nutrition recommendations on carbohydrates, including sugars and fibre.* https://www.gov.uk/government/publications/sacn-carbohydrates-and-health-report. Accessed 20 Jan 2019.

Stewart, H. (2016). *George Osborne backs sugar tax and £3.5bn of Whitehall cuts* [Online]. Available: https://www.theguardian.com/uk-news/2016/mar/16/george-osbornes-sugar-tax-economic-fears-budget. Accessed 2 Feb 2019.

Sugar Association Letter to WHO, A. (2003, April). Sugar Association Letter to WHO. http://www.documentcloud.org/documents/458188-sugar-association-letter-to-who-april-2003.html. Accessed 22 Dec 2018.

Te Morenga, L., Mallard, S., & Mann, J. (2013). Dietary sugars and body weight: Systematic review and meta-analyses of randomised controlled trials and cohort studies. *BMJ, 346*, E7492.

Tedstone, A., Targett, V., & Allen, R. (2015). *Sugar reduction: The evidence for action.* https://assets.publishing.service.gov.uk/government/uploads/system/uploads/attachment_data/file/470179/Sugar_reduction_The_evidence_for_action.pdf. Accessed 10 Feb 2019.

WHO. (2003). *Diet, nutrition and the prevention of chronic diseases* [Online]. Available: http://www.fao.org/docrep/005/AC911E/ac911e00.htm. Accessed 2 Feb 2019.

WHO. (2014). *The science behind the sweetness in our diets* [Online]. Available: https://www.who.int/bulletin/volumes/92/11/14-031114/en/. Accessed 6 Feb 2019.

WHO. (2015). *WHO calls on countries to reduce sugars intake among adults and children* [Online]. Available: https://www.who.int/mediacentre/news/releases/2015/sugar-guideline/en/. Accessed 2 Feb 2019.

WHO. (2019). *Childhood overweight and obesity* [Online]. Available: https://www.who.int/dietphysicalactivity/childhood/en/. Accessed 2 Feb 2019.

Yudkin, J. (1988). *Pure, white and deadly.* London: Penguin.

CHAPTER 7

The Policy Evaluation Risk Communication Framework

THE POLICY EVALUATION RISK COMMUNICATION FRAMEWORK

The analysis of the smoking, MMR vaccine and sugar safety debates was carried out through the lens of the PERC framework to understand how power and expertise shape public health risk discussion in the policy domain. The PERC framework is based on the assumption that *social amplification of risk drives the negotiation of public health risk argument such that an argument becomes dominant in a policy domain*. The analysis also suggests that social amplification of risk is a multi-dimensional and multi-channel process (Fischbacher-Smith 2012). The PERC framework illustrates how power, expertise, communication and trust shape risk communication about public health and safety. However, emphasis is placed on the role of power and expertise and how these interact to shape public debate about public health and safety. The PERC framework highlights several hidden yet salient dimensions of power that shape the multi-dimensionality of social amplification of risk in risk debates. These are non-decision-making power, ideological power, stakeholders relationships, tactics of domination (legislation, punishment) and resistance (counter-arguments), and the wider societal context including historic events and future uncertainty.

The following section examines the findings of the smoking, MMR vaccine and sugar debates through the lens of the PERC framework and then critically analyses these within the context of extant literature.

Smoking Debate Through the PERC Framework

The result of the evolving events within the UK smoking debate (between 1950 and 1998) shows that the main thrust of the debate centred on: (a) the nature of evidence (which was largely statistical) linking smoking tobacco and lung cancer; (b) how the evidence should be framed within the public health context and (c) disagreements about precautionary measures put in place to mitigate the dangers of smoking to health. In the UK, the smoking debate emerged following Doll and Hill's (1950) study in which they suggested that there was statistical association between smoking tobacco and lung cancer. This suggestion puts the burden of proof on the shoulders of the tobacco industry, as well as public health institutions or officials charged with the responsibility of communicating and informing the public of the health risks they face. In this book, the smoking debate is examined in three phases. The first period covered between 1950 and 1955, the second period covered the smoking debate between 1956 and 1965, and the third period examined the unfolding events between 966 and 1998.

In the first phase, analysis of the evolving events suggests that evidence linking smoking tobacco and lung cancer was in its embryonic state at this point and the initial debate centred on the nature of evidence. Although at this point public health officials accepted Doll and Hill's publication, they were cautious of the nature of the evidence. This is clear in a memo written to the Cabinet Home Affairs Committee, where the then Minister of Health noted that "there is no precise evidence of how tobacco smoking causes cancer of the lung". However, he accepted that there was a convincing argument for an association between tobacco smoking and lung cancer. Associates of the tobacco industry at this early stage can be seen to be seeking out public trust when they said, "if it should ever be proved that there exists something harmful in tobacco... [They] will be the first to act ..." (Chairman of Imperial Tobacco Statement 1953). In addition, they rejected and challenged the technical case made against smoking (highlighting weaknesses and gaps in existing knowledge). Within this period, the government took no steps or initiative to mitigate smoking risk. This initial lack of response from the government can be linked to many factors, including the fact that smoking was considered a normal activity, and also the statistical nature of the evidence, but it may also be for economic reasons that the government ignored the dangers of smoking. Similar studies have also raised other potential reasons, including electoral concerns over interfering in mass public behaviour and the dangers of creating further pressure over the air pollution debate in the 1950s (Berridge 2006).

With reference to the PERC framework, power, expertise, communication and trust can be seen to shape the smoking debate within this period. In terms of power, both non-decision-making power and agency and structure seem to be relevant here. Non-decision-making power is seen in the ability of the MRC and Ministry of Health to put the smoking risk issue on the public health agenda in the 1950s. The consideration of lung cancer and its relationship to smoking cigarettes led to the sponsorship of Doll and Hill's research, which raised awareness of and triggered the direction of the debate on the risk to health from smoking in such a way that smoking policy became a public health priority. Giddens' (1979) perspective on power can be observed in the pattern of stakeholders' (social/professional) relationships. In this case, there was a professional relationship between technical experts (such as Doll and Hill) and policymakers, which allowed for contact and exchange of views that brought about hegemony within government departments as early as the mid-1950s of a risk discourse in which smoking is linked to lung cancer.

In terms of expertise, technical 'expertise' was the means by which public health officials made sense of rising incidences of lung cancer, and the role of smoking was made explicit through technical experts' interpretation of evidence (even if it was only statistical in nature). The interpretation of a 'real association' between smoking tobacco and lung cancer would have resonated with policymakers, and the manner in which they responded by accepting this association signifies the importance of technical expertise in policy inquiry and policy development relating to risk. In addition, the policy perspective of government departments of public health was aided by the advice and recommendations of expert technical committees and advisory bodies. This observation is in line with the view that sees science and its experts as a sense-making aid to risk issues within the policy domain (Collingridge and Reeve 1986; Jasanoff 1996; Fischbacher-Smith 2012).

It is also important to note how the tobacco industry demanded causal (biological) proof that links smoking of tobacco cigarettes and lung cancer. Highlighting this uncertainty and these gaps in knowledge created doubt in the public consciousness and raised questions about the validity of the technical case against smoking and its relation to lung cancer. It could also have been a way to divert attention from the real health concerns associated with smoking. Trust and credibility also seem to be pertinent here as relevant public health authorities such as the CHSC and SACCR accepted Doll and Hill's interpretations and urged the government to create public awareness of the dangers of smoking. This acceptance was an indication of trust in the credibility of Doll and Hill's conclusions. This was also captured in the words of Dr. Green, who, after a meeting between a representative of the tobacco companies and Richard Hill, expressed the view that "It was pretty clear to me that Mr Partridge and his colleagues felt that Hill had answered all their queries in a way which left hardly any loophole for doubt…" (ash.org.uk). Representatives of the tobacco industry also understood the importance of trust when they demanded public trust in their corporate social responsibilities.

The second phase of the smoking debate (between 1956 and 1966) analysed in this book saw the state of scientific evidence evolve from an embryonic one. Evidence at this stage (although still largely statistical) continued to link smoking tobacco and lung cancer. It was in this period that the industry heightened its demand for a causal link. Using its own technical experts, the industry launched a fierce attack on the technical case made against smoking. The industry offered £250,000 for research to the MRC, stating that a link between smoking tobacco and lung cancer can only be proven "when medical science is able to provide a causal proof to the claim" (Statement Issued by the Group of Leading Tobacco Manufacturers 1954). The government response within this period was initially aimed at educating and informing the public of the dangers of smoking. This saw the establishment of the Health Education Council (HEC). The HEC was later reorganised as the Health Education Authority in Scotland, England and Wales.

Other competing hypotheses also emerged at this point questioning the validity of the case linking smoking tobacco and lung cancer (Berkson 1958; Fisher 1959; Hueper 1956; Berkson 1955). These critics point to environmental factors and factors other than smoking that might predispose an individual to lung cancer, for instance genotype (Fisher 1958). Fisher (1958) argued that an individual 'gene' may predispose such a person to both 'smoking' and 'cancer'. However, such alternative arguments (e.g. environmental factors and the genetic argument) received little attention in the policy domain. The technical case linking tobacco to lung cancer was boosted following pressure from elite groups, personalities and public health experts for stricter tobacco control by the government.

With reference to the PERC framework, communication (in terms of the language in use) featured very strongly at this point in shaping the smoking debate. Public health authorities can be seen to use negative frames to qualify the dangers of smoking to health, including "mortality from cancer of the lung is twenty times greater amongst heavy smokers than amongst non-smokers"; "the most reasonable interpretation of scientific evidence is that the relationship is one of direct cause and effect" and "the most credible interpretation and explanation for the increase in the death of cancer of the lung". These frames signify that public health authorities accepted the suggestion that smoking was in fact dangerous to public health and safety. Representatives of the tobacco industry continued to use language of uncertainty in the continuing controversy and to dismiss the technical case made against smoking. They called for more research before any causal association could be established.

By using language of uncertainty, representatives of the industry continually highlighted uncertainties and gaps in scientific knowledge. They used frames such as "conflicting and incomplete" (Statement By A Group of Leading Tobacco Manufacturers in the UK 1956); "there is no proof" (Partridge 1956); "it has not been established with any certainty" (Tobacco Manufacturers' Standing Committee 1957); "no conclusive proofs" (McCormick 1962) and "the mechanisms of these diseases are not understood" (TMDP 1990). The use of language of uncertainty undermined the validity of the claim that smoking is related to lung cancer for some time, until evidence began to tilt the balance of power away from the tobacco industry. This also created doubt in the minds of the public and may also have been a strategic move to divert attention from the real dangers of smoking to health. This discourse of causal proof or causality was corroborated by Dr. Green, the head of the BAT research unit, in his paper titled "Cigarette Smoking and Causal Relationships". He noted that

> The industry has retreated behind impossible demands for 'scientific proof' whereas such proof has never been required as a basis for action in the legal and political fields ... It may therefore be concluded that for certain groups of people smoking causes the incidence of certain diseases to be higher than it would otherwise be. (Green 1976)

The discourse of causal proof, or the causality frame used by the tobacco industry, became a lens through which the industry highlighted the uncertainties surrounding the claim that smoking is linked to lung cancer. It also acted as a barrier to timely and appropriate policy interventions; even at this time there had been no concrete policy interventions. In addition, the discourse of causal proof served to protect the principles of CSR and accountability because until the industry accepted an association between smoking tobacco and lung cancer, it would be wrong for it to be acting in a manner that could be seen as socially irresponsible. Besides the discourse of causal proof used by representatives of the tobacco industry, another narrative they used was the notion of 'moderation'. They used frames such as "Neither tobacco, nor alcohol is harmful, in moderation" (BBC panorama TV 1962) and "Anything can be considered harmful. Apple sauce is harmful if you get too much of it" (Thames Television 1976).

In terms of power and expertise in this phase, the establishment of the TMSC increased the industry's influence and ability to exercise power over the production of scientific evidence and its interpretation.

The last phase of the smoking debate examined (the period between 1966 and 1998) saw a slow but gradual implementation of initiatives to mitigate smoking risk from both the tobacco industry and departments of public health. This was initially through voluntary agreement between the government and the industry on how tobacco should be promoted and sold. It signified a shift in the tobacco industry's power strategy, from one of attacking the technical case made against smoking, to one focusing on efforts towards influencing policy developments relating to mitigating the risk of smoking. This change of strategy perhaps can be linked to the evolved state of evidence linking tobacco to lung cancer and how this is influencing the nature of argument brought to bear on the debate. The governance response was initially aimed at educating the public, leading to organisations such as the HEC in England, Wales and Scotland and Action on Smoking and Health (ASH) being set up to educate the public and de-glamourise smoking in society (ash.org.uk). Subsequently, more concrete and binding action was put into place, including the enactment of the Children and Young Persons (Protection from Tobacco) Act 1991 that increased penalties to anyone selling tobacco products to children under the age of 16 years. There was also the ban on tobacco advertising in the UK and EU under the European Union's Directive (ash.org.uk). What can also be observed was the shift in the language used by public health authorities in characterising the dangers of smoking. This saw a shift from the use of a language of uncertainty to one of certainty.

In terms of the PERC framework, Giddens' (1979) notion of structural power exercised by means of social relationships was particularly significant here. Through voluntary agreement, the industry negotiated a television advertisement ban before 9:00 pm (Collingridge and Reeve 1986) and negotiated ways of raising public awareness about the dangers of smoking tobacco cigarettes, including warnings on cigarette packs and developing tobacco substitutes (Collingridge and Reeve 1986). These negotiations strengthened the industry's political position by enabling it to delay or make unnecessary the establishment of stricter and legally binding rules. For example, the 1971 negotiation over health warnings on tobacco products (accepted by the government) meant that there was no need for a Private Bill in the House of Commons which demanded a much stronger warning on cigarette packs (Popham 1981).

Voluntary agreement also gave the industry more insight into the government position on smoking, enabling it to make more strategic arguments relating to smoking policy. Because of its economic power the tobacco industry was also able to circumvent the advertising ban in the UK, thereby undermining the message that smoking is a danger to public health, by sharply increasing its sponsorship of sporting and cultural events. In some cases, this involved racing cars bearing the names of cigarettes that could not be advertised (WHO report, 2013). The industry also used loopholes in the law to delay, restrict or influence government policies on tobacco control. For example, in 1991, the UK tobacco industry sued the UK government over the size of the new health warnings that were to be printed on cigarette packs.

Evidence also suggests that the industry attempted to influence policy through its network of advisors. For example, a BBC Panorama programme found that one of the members of the sport council was the chairperson of the Tobacco Advisory Council. The presence of an ally in the sport council meant that the interest of the tobacco industry was potentially protected in the policy advice given to the government on sporting issues. It also enhanced its ability to gain insight into policy thinking that might advantage its strategic positioning. The change of tobacco industry strategy was adequately captured by the words of Dr. Jim Green, in an interview after his retirement as the head of the BAT research unit, with which he served for 20 years:

At the beginning of the sixties the tobacco companies realized there was serious evidence connecting smoking and ill health. Their first reaction was to spend money on research to see if this was true, in the hope that it wasn't, so they could win the argument. When this failed, the research effort was directed to finding a safe cigarette, through the development of substitutes. When this flopped in the mid-seventies there was a sharp change of direction. New, corporate careerists were now in charge of the companies and they had fewer qualms about the business they were in; research was redirected to serve the interests of marketing. This development coalesced rather well with the attitude that the companies had taken towards the health risk and regulation policy. On the advice of their PR man, they pursued a 'tight-rope' policy on health ... and entered into voluntary agreements because this bought them time. (Green 1972, ash.org.uk)

The analysis of the evolving events also reveals that there are negative and real consequences associated with the excessive exercise of power (as exemplified by the tobacco industry) in risk communication about public health and safety and associated policymaking. First, excessive exercise of power may lead to a delay in policy interventions, which may result in taking either over-precautionary or under-precautionary measures. In the smoking debate, the excessive exercise of power by the tobacco industry (made possible by its resources) led to delays in the appropriate policy interventions. This is evidenced by the fact that the first policy White Paper on tobacco control was presented to Parliament in 1998 despite an awareness of the dangers of smoking and a seeming consensus in government departments from as early as the mid-1950s. The absence of any concrete smoking-mitigating strategy over this long span of time undermined the smoking/cancer argument, thereby exposing the public to the risk of smoking for much longer than it should have been.

MMR Through the Lens of the PERC Framework

The main thrust of the MMR vaccine debate centred on whether the institutionalised MMR vaccine immunisation routine was safe for young infants given its suggested link to autism. Andrew Wakefield and his colleagues at the Royal Free Hospital in 1998 suggested that there was an association between the MMR vaccine and autism, and called for a precautionary approach to use a single injection until any risk from the MMR vaccine was ruled out. However, this unproven hypothesis linking MMR vaccine and autism was fiercely opposed by public health officials responsible for public health and safety.

While some of the co-authors retracted their support for the 1998 paper, Wakefield insisted for many years that the MMR vaccine was unsafe for some young infants. He claimed in several studies that the MMR vaccine had not undergone suitable safety tests. Within the first phase of the debate, public health institutions responsible for advising the UK government on routine immunisation, such as the DoH, the Committee on Safety of Medicines, the MCA and the JCVI were quick to dismiss Wakefield's claims, accusing him of cherry-picking evidence, unethical conduct and committing fraudulent acts. These authorities argued that the triple MMR vaccine was safe and preferable to single-component injections (Bosley 2001). No policy changes were recommended or made in the first analysed phase of the debate.

The second phase of the debate (2001 and 2003) showed that Wakefield continued to insist that the MMR vaccine was unsafe for young infants (Fraser 2001). This period also saw a rise in measles outbreaks in the UK. At this point, the government, realising the importance of communication and trust between public and health authorities, launched a £3 million advertising campaign in order to cope with a growing concern about the use of the triple MMR vaccination (Boseley 2001). Public health authorities continued to criticise Wakefield's conduct but also argued that giving combined doses of MMR vaccines was safer than administering them individually (DoH 2001). In addition, the Brian Deer investigation revealed that Wakefield received research aid of over £50,000 from a legal team working against vaccine manufacturers (Deer 2004). While Wakefield disclosed that there was a link between himself and the Legal Aid Board which was sent to *The Lancet* three months before his 1998 publication in that journal (Booth 2004), he did not mention the money he was paid for the study. He was removed from the British medical register by the General Medical Council on account of serious professional misconduct in 2010 (Meikle and Boseley 2010).

Giddens' (1979) notion of structural power manifested through stakeholder relationships seems to be significant here in shaping the policy perspective taken to risk. This was manifest in the stakeholder relationship between policymakers and technical experts (the 37-member expert committee) whose expertise was called upon to make sense of the risk to public health. The committee recommended no change to the then MMR vaccine programme and this led to the policy conclusion that the MMR vaccine was indeed safe and in the best interest of infants and public health. Wakefield's membership of the medical profession gave him the authority and mandate to speak to this domain of risk, which, combined with his statement or explanation which was open to interpretation in the press conference following the first publication of his findings, may have also sparked the public controversy over whether the MMR vaccine is linked to autism.

Foucault's notion of resistive power can be observed in terms of some parents' refusal to give consent to their infants being given the MMR vaccine, and opting instead for the single immunisation components (Evans et al. 2001). This was evidenced in the significant reduction in the uptake of the MMR vaccine to below the threshold of herd immunity for the first time since the introduction of the vaccine. Parents' exercise of resistive power led the government to change its communication strategy from giving reassurance to a two-way and interactive one through the launch of a new website: "MMR: The facts". The aim of the website was to raise awareness about the significance of the MMR vaccine and to act as an information source for parents who needed updates on the continuing controversy.

The MMR vaccine debate can be seen to be largely influenced by technical experts from its inception. This controversy began when Wakefield suggested that there was potentially a link between the MMR vaccine and autism despite his study not proving any relationship. Certainly, it was his suggestion of a possible link in a press statement on the eve of the publication and subsequent media presentation that raised the concerns of parents who were looking to make the safest choices for their children. Technical experts, for example the 37-member expert committee, can also be seen to act as policy advisers advising the government on the policy action in the interest of public health. For example, their conclusion not to change the MMR vaccine policy programme encouraged government officials to quickly refute Wakefield's claims and reassure concerned parents that MMR vaccine policy was indeed safe for both infants and the general wellbeing of the public.

The first examined phase of the MMR vaccine debate also illustrates the bias against experiential expertise, which is undervalued in fields of contested knowledge. This can be seen in parents' observations linking the start of changes to their children's behavioural responses to the MMR vaccination. Nevertheless, the fear-mongering discourse of Andrew Wakefield linking the MMR vaccine and autism, combined with some of the parents' accounts of their children's behavioural changes, may have amplified risk (erroneously) in the face of scientific evidence.

With reference to communication and trust, what seems apparent is how the government's initial response was focused on reassuring parents that the claim that the MMR vaccine was linked to autism was unsubstantiated. However, these reassurances were carried out in a one-way communication fashion that is now recognised as a deficient model for risk communication about public health and safety. This perhaps may be one reason why MMR vaccine uptake was found to have declined in some parts of the country, despite quick government reassurance. This suggested that the government's official reassurances that the MMR vaccine was safe failed to convince some concerned parents in some parts of the UK. However, there was another study that blamed the decline of MMR vaccine uptake on media scares (Anderson 1999). Subsequently, the launching of the website enabled a forum for parents to ask questions directly to members of the DoH, a move towards a more two-way communication.

The Sugar Debate Through the PERC Framework

The core contention around the sugar debate centred on the suggested link between high sugar consumption and weight gain and the implication this has for the different age groups of the public, especially children. Obesity has been identified as a major public health issue and sugar is seen as a major contributing factor to obesity, which in turn increases risk of a number of heart diseases and other conditions including dental caries. Obesity, for example, is said to cost the NHS over £5 billion annually, and as a consequence risk reduction measures have been put in place to reduce sugar consumption in the UK, including the contentious soft drink industry levy, following the established evidence that sugar is linked to obesity (Te Morenga et al. 2013).

With regard to the PERC framework, analysis of the sugar debate shows that the WHO was a key influential agent in shaping the research agenda and in the arguments brought to bear on the sugar debate through its several commissioned studies. For example, in 2003, the WHO recommended a 10% reduction in sugar in dietary intake. This recommendation was set out following the call by the WHO to investigate the link between sugar and body weight (Boseley 2003). By so doing, the WHO, and other public health organisations such as Public Health England, can be seen to exercise non-decision making (by shaping the sugar research agenda).

The analysis of the tobacco debate also shows that various *ideological* mechanisms were used by the sugar industry to shape public acceptability of the sugar debate. For example, the industry was quick to stress the economic importance of sugar through job creation and sugar tax. There were also arguments about the 'nanny state' where critics of the sugar tax questioned the effectiveness of this tax to curb obesity, an assessment shared by the then government for a while until evidence began to shift this held view. Instead, the argument to focus on physical activity and individual responsibility was put forward.

The analysis of the sugar debate also shows powerful influence of stakeholder relationships in influencing the sugar debate. For example, there existed a relationship between public health institution and expert groups (e.g. the WHO and the 37-member expert committee), between the industry and their expert groups (Public Health England and its expert committee) and between public health institutions. The WHO, for example, can be seen to be influential at the international level and this influence can be seen to shape the decision-making process at the national level. In the UK, for example, the UK medical community following the WHO revised its recommendations, urging the government to adopt WHO recommendations. WHO influence at the international level, combined with the backing of many public health organisations (e.g. SACN, *PHE*) and public groups (and celebrities such as Jamie Oliver), can be said to have pressured the UK government to change its childhood obesity reduction strategy, evident in their narrative of "more effective ways of tackling obesity" to a surprise announcement of a sugar tax in 2016. This suggests that while there is a direct stakeholder relationship (e.g. between policymakers and expert committee), a less direct stakeholder relationship (through discourse coalition) can be a powerful mechanism that shapes the risk acceptability debate and its regulation. One benefit of stakeholder relationships for the sugar industry was that it enabled the concept of voluntary agreement and self-regulation to flourish for a while until the sugar legislation came into effect in 2018.

There was also a counter-argument that suggests that resistance as a form of power was also expressed in the sugar debate. The sugar industry can be seen to attack the technical case made against smoking and point to evidence where possible to support its worldview, for example, following the study published by the University of Cambridge linking 8000 cases of type 2 diabetes to sugar consumption (Imamura et al. 2015). Gavin Partington, British Soft Drinks Association, was quick to assert that there was insufficient evidence on an international level to make any conclusive evidence (Boseley 2016).

Technical experts were key influential agents in the sugar debate. For example, Simon Stevens, Chief Executive of NHS England, likened the obesity problem to "the new smoking" challenge (Campbell 2015), whilst the WHO describes this as one of the top challenges to public health in the twenty-first century (WHO 2019). Likening the sugar issue to the tobacco debate again raised the issue of trust around the ability of industry, who enjoy economic benefit, to make decisions in the best interest of public health before any private gains. Thus, the entrenched mistrust from the smoking debate can be seen to be fairly important in the sugar debate.

Having analysed the three case studies (smoking, MMR vaccine and sugar debates), it can be seen that the PERC framework is relevant and able to explain how certain perspectives of risk become amplified and how risk arguments transition between over-critical and under-critical models in the policy context. Nevertheless, further empirical research is needed to validate how behavioural response to policy interventions may shape the transition between over-critical and under-critical models. The analysis of the tobacco and sugar debates (where the burden of proof lies on an industry) found that similar tactics were used by the tobacco and sugar industries as the debate evolved and as evidence emerged. For example, the tobacco and sugar industries can be seen to change their power strategy from one of attacking the technical case made against smoking/sugar and lung cancer/obesity by means of technical expertise, to focusing effort on influencing policy development relating to smoking using professional lobbyists and government allies. The analysis of the two debates showed that this shift occurred as a result of the evolved state of evidence, information and knowledge that tilted the balance of power against the tobacco and sugar industries in the two respective debates.

Analysis of the three debates also shows that that there is a strong relation between the ability of stakeholder groups to exercise power (amplified by economic resources) and social amplification (or attenuation) in public health risk communication and its associated policymaking. Industries with economic power (such as tobacco and the sugar industries) are able to use the economic resources within their means to

(a) purchase the necessary technical expertise to shape risk debates; (b) enhance trust through scientific credibility; (c) control communication by means of language used and (d) influence policy processes by means of stakeholder relationships. Such power has been expressed by either defining policy priorities or determining whose expertise is called upon and whose questions are asked in the technical analysis of risk. There was also legitimate power expressed through laws that prohibit the sale of tobacco to the underaged and restrictions on tobacco sale and advertisement. In addition is resistive power that was expressed through boycotts and bans on smoking in public and office spaces. Against this background, *'power' in risk communication about public health and safety within its policy context may be expressed through technical expertise, control of communication and creation or destruction of trust (through scientific activities).*

Furthermore, the analysis of the tobacco and sugar debates (analysed in this book) and the EC debate (analysed in Adekola et al. 2018) shows some emerging trends around the shift in policy regulation as the state of evidence, information and knowledge evolves in a risk debate.

Table 7.1 describes this shifting policy regulation in an evolving risk debate. In the early phases of risk debates, typically characterised by little and emerging evidence that implicates certain practices, there is the tendency to have self-regulation and voluntary agreement between the associated industry and policymakers. When this evidence evolves, mounting further evidence and implicating this source of hazard, self or voluntary

Table 7.1 The transition of policy regulation in an evolving risk debate

State of evidence/policy and industry response	Emerging state of a risk debate (little or no evidence/ unknown)	Evolved state of evidence (known unknown)	Mature state of understanding of risk
Policy regulation	Self-regulation and voluntary arrangement	Emerging legislation: Initial development and emergence of legally binding policy regulation.	Legislation extension: Extending the boundaries of initial regulation and institutionalising the regulation
Industry power strategy response	Attack on the technical case made against product/services.	Lobbying and developing new technologies around regulation.	Adhering to policy regulation or a change of business strategy.

regulation tends to shift to a soft regulation. The boundary of this soft regulation is then shifted to a hard regulation as the full consequences of the risk are understood. The transition between the three phases of policy regulation is a two-way process as the successes or emergent problems from policy regulation may mean that policy regulation is rolled back. It is the contention of this book that the nature of power and expertise brought to bear on the risk debate by the different stakeholder groups determines how quickly we transition through the different policy regulation phases.

REFERENCES

1954. Statement issued by a group of leading tobacco manufacturers in the UK.
Action on Smoking and Health. (2017). Key dates in the history of anti-tobacco campaigning. http://ash.org.uk/information-and-resources/briefings/key-datesin-the-history-of-anti-tobacco-campaigning/. Accessed 2 June 2016.
Adekola, J., Fischbacher-Smith, D., & Fischbacher-Smith, M. (2018). Light me up: Power and expertise in risk communication and policy-making in the e-cigarette health debates. *Journal of Risk Research*, 1–15.
Anderson, P. (1999). Another media scare about MMR vaccine hits Britain. *BMJ, 318*, 1578.
ash.org.uk. *Smoking and health* [Online]. Available: http://webcache.googleusercontent.com/search?q=cache:WvSGWd55fd0J:www.ash.org.uk/files/documents/ASH_99.pdf+&cd=1&hl=en&ct=clnk&gl=uk. Accessed 07 July 2016.
BBC Panorama programme reports on the tobacco industry, 1962. Directed by BBC.
Berkson, J. (1955). The statistical study of association between smoking and lung cancer. *Proceedings of Staff Meetings of the Mayo Clinic, 30*(15), 319–348.
Berkson, J. (1958). Smoking and lung cancer: Some observations on two recent reports. *Journal of the American Statistical Association, 53*, 28–38.
Berridge, V. (2006). The policy response to the smoking and lung cancer connection in the 1950s and 1960s. *Historical Journal-London-Cambridge University Press, 49*, 1185.
Booth, J. (2004). MMR jabs doctor declared interest. https://www.theguardian.com/uk/2004/feb/27/highereducation.science. Accessed 18 May 2016.
Boseley, S. (2001). Doctor's green light for MMR campaign. https://www.theguardian.com/society/2001/nov/20/publichealth. Accessed 8 May 2016.
Boseley, S. (2003). *Sugar industry threatens to scupper WHO* [Online]. Available: https://www.theguardian.com/society/2003/apr/21/usnews.food. Accessed 2 Feb 2019.
Boseley, S. (2016). *Price of sugary soft drinks could rise by 8p a can when tax introduced* [Online]. Available: https://www.theguardian.com/lifeandstyle/2016/dec/05/price-of-sugary-soft-drinks-could-rise-by-8p-a-can-when-tax-introduced. Accessed 2 Feb 2019.

Bosley, S. (2001, January 23). Alternative to MMR jab 'not safe'. *The Guardian*.
Campbell, D. (2015, July 13). Government delays publication of plans for reduction in UK'S sugar intake. *The Guardian*.
Collingridge, D., & Reeve, C. (1986). *Science speaks to power: The role of experts in policy making*. London: Francis Pinter.
Committee, T. M. S. 1957. Smoking and Lung Cancer. https://www.theguardian.com/theguardian/2010/jun/28/archive-one-in-eight-of-heavy-smokers-doomed-1957
Death in the West, 1976. Directed by Television, T.
Deer, B. (2004). MMR: The truth behind the crisis. *Sunday Times*.
DoH, M. A. (2001). Combined measles, mumps and rubella vaccines: Response of the Medicines Control Agency and Department of Health to issues raised in papers published in *Adverse drug reactions and toxicological reviews*.
Doll, R., & Hill, B. (1950). Smoking and carcinoma of the lung; preliminary report. *British Medical Journal, 2*, 739–748.
Evans, M., Stoddart, H., Condon, L., Freeman, E., Grizzell, M., & Mullen, R. (2001). Parents' perspectives on the MMR immunisation: A focus group study. *The British Journal of General Practice, 51*, 904–910.
Fischbacher-Smith, D. (2012). Getting pandas to breed: Paradigm blindness and the policy space for risk prevention, mitigation and management. *Risk Management, 14*, 177–201.
Fisher, R. A. (1958). Lung cancer and cigarettes? *Nature, 182*, 108.
Fisher, S. R. A. (1959). *Smoking: The cancer controversy: Some attempts to assess the evidence*. Edinburgh: Oliver and Boyd London.
Fraser, L. (2001, January 21). MMR doctor links 170 cases of autism to vaccine. *The Telegraph Newspaper*.
Giddens, A. (1979). Agency, structure. In *Central problems in social theory* (pp. 49–95). London: Palgrave.
Gilliam, A. G. (1955). Trends of mortality attributed to carcinoma of the lung: Possible effects of faulty certification of deaths to other respiratory diseases. *Cancer, 8*, 1130–1136.
Green, S. (1972). Safety evaluation of cigarettes. Pollock 67.
Green, S. (1975). Basis for research in smoking. Pollock 56.
Green, SJ. (1976). Cigarette smoking and causal relationships. 27 October 1976—Internet Ref. 2331.08. Cited in Pollock, D., 1996. Forty years on: A war to recognise and win: How the tobacco industry has survived the revelations on smoking and health. *British Medical Bulletin, 52*(1), 174–182.
Hueper, W. (1956). A quest into the environmental causes of cancer of the lung. *Public Health Monograph*.
Imamura, F., O'connor, L., Ye, Z., Mursu, J., Hayashino, Y., Bhupathiraju, S. N., & Forouhi, N. G. (2015). Consumption of sugar sweetened beverages, artificially sweetened beverages, and fruit juice and incidence of type 2 diabetes:

Systematic review, meta-analysis, and estimation of population attributable fraction. *BMJ, 351*, h3576.

Jasanoff, S. (1996). Beyond epistemology: Relativism and engagement in the politics of science. *Social Studies of Science, 26*, 393–418.

Manufacturers, U. T. (1956). Statement by a group of leading tobacco manufacturers in the UK. http://news.bbc.co.uk/onthisday/hi/dates/stories/may/7/newsid_2518000/2518245.stm.

McCormick, A. (1962). Smoking and health: Policy on research. In Minutes of Southampton Meeting.

Meikle, J., & Boseley, S. (2010). MMR row doctor Andrew Wakefield struck off register. *The Guardian*.

Partridge, E. J. (1956, March 9). *RE: Letter from representative of tobacco industry to Sir John Hawton*. Type to Hawton, S. J.

Popham, G. T. (1981). Government and smoking: Policy-making and pressure groups. *Policy & Politics, 9*, 331–348.

Te Morenga, L., Mallard, S., & Mann, J. (2013). Dietary sugars and body weight: Systematic review and meta-analyses of randomised controlled trials and cohort studies. *BMJ, 346*, e7492.

TMDP. (1990). A talk given by a Senior BAT Executive at Chelwood. In R. O. T. T. Industry (Ed.). https://www.industrydocuments.ucsf.edu/tobacco/docs/#id=lgfw0200.

Tobacco, C. O. I. (1953, March 17). *RE: The Chairman of Imperial Tobacco to Shareholders*. Type to Shareholders.

WHO. (2019). *Childhood overweight and obesity* [Online]. Available: https://www.who.int/dietphysicalactivity/childhood/en/. Accessed 2 Feb 2019.

CHAPTER 8

The Role of Power and Expertise in Social Amplification of Risk

WEAKNESS IN THE EXISTING CONCEPTUALISATION OF SARF

In Chap. 3 of this book, a critical review of the SARF led to the identification of several weaknesses. Within this, it was observed that the SARF over-emphasised the 'who' factor (i.e. sources, channels and transmitters), especially 'the media', in amplifying (or attenuating) risk signals. While this is valuable, it ignores underlying factors such as power and expertise that condition the amplification (or attenuation) process of risk, especially in the information mechanism stage of the SARF. It is on this basis that the alternative perspective of the SARF is presented here. This account of the SARF is built rather on the assumption that social amplification of risk is a multi-channel and multi-dimensional process (Fischbacher-Smith 2012). This perspective recognises the dynamic representations of the different stakeholder groups (Pidgeon et al. 2003) and makes a radical move away from the view that sees the media as the primary amplifier. The assumption here is that scientific experts and the science they know, understand and communicate are powerful influences that may thereafter form the basis of debate, mediated by the other groups (including the media). This suggests that social amplification of risk may even occur before it reaches the overt risk arena, as a result of expert technical identification, construction and communication of the risk. This assumption is in line with the views of Irwin (2015), who argued that there is a recurrent predisposition among political, regulatory and scientific institutions (charged with the responsibilities of managing the risk) to separate the processes of knowledge production and risk communication.

Power and Social Amplification of Risk

The analysis of the smoking, MMR vaccine and sugar debates suggests that there are multiple dimensions by which social amplification (or attenuation) of risk may occur.

Non-decision-making Power in Risk Debate

The smoking, MMR vaccine and sugar debates as analysed in this book showed that non-decision-making power (Bachrach and Baratz 1962) was able to explain how certain stakeholder groups can exercise the "non-decision making" (p. 952) power and how this shaped risk communication about public health and safety. For example, the evolving events in the smoking risk debate suggest that the MRC and Ministry of Health exercised non-decision-making power by prioritising inquiry into the relationship between smoking tobacco and lung cancer in the 1950s. This consideration led to the sponsorship of Doll and Hill's research that triggered the emergence of the smoking debate, making smoking risk a health priority in the UK. The same exercise of non-decision-making power applies to public health authorities that determined what questions were essential in assessing the incorrect suggestion that the MMR vaccine was linked to autism. There were those who were interested in understanding the causes of autism. Instead, initial emphasis of the 37-expert committee conveyed by the Minister of Health focused on examining (validating or refuting) Andrew Wakefield's evidence. Non-decision-making power was also expressed by the WHO and then Public Health England about the risk of sugar, which raised concerns about the relationship between sugar and weight gain/obesity and poor dental health. Following this inquiry, these organisations recommended a 10% and 5% limit on dietary sugar intake respectively.

Such non-decision-making power as exercised by public health authorities (seen in the smoking, MMR vaccine and sugar case studies) influenced the initial direction and scope of the discussion, which prevented any overt conflicts or initial challenges from other stakeholder groups. This finding is similar to Birkland (2017), who suggested that setting the risk or policy agenda determines which risk issue or solution gains public and policy attention, which will ultimately drive the issue and, conversely, reduce the significance of those issues or problems relating to the risk that fail to make it on to the agenda. Bachrach and Baratz (1962) raised caution about the ways policymakers define 'critical' or 'key' issues that make an issue a policy priority. They argue for a "restrictive face of power" that considers non-decision making, and which can be used: (a) to uncover procedural, institutional or social bias and the extent to which powerful persons and groups are able to influence those values and institutions that are brought to bear in risk communication and that may profit or disadvantage certain groups; (b) as a foundation for analysing those directly or indirectly involved in decision-making; and (c) as processes that differentiate between 'key' and 'routine' policy decisions. Bachrach and Baratz (1962) reject any suggestion that undermines this as a useful means of deconstructing non-decision-making power in risk discussion, despite recognising that identifying these restrictive or enabling forces is a subjective act.

Ideological Power in Risk Debate

Ideological power – the capacity to influence others in a covert way – can also be seen to be manifest in the analysis of the evolving events relating to the smoking, MMR vaccine and sugar debates. Ideological power was expressed through technical expertise and media sources, which are the means by which interested stakeholders and the public made sense of the risks they face. For example, the expert interpretation that links smoking tobacco and lung cancer expressed by Doll and Hill was accepted by key government advisory bodies, and this interpretation shaped the policy perspective taken on smoking risk. In the sugar debate, ideological power can be seen to be exercised by public health organisations, technical expertise and pressure groups (e.g. Jamie Oliver's Sugar Rush documentary) to shape public and policy understanding of the scale of the sugar problem and the need for an urgent response.

Ideological power can also be observed in the MMR vaccine safety debate where Andrew Wakefield suggested a potential link between the MMR vaccine and autism. His assertion created a lot of tension and distress in relation to public health and safety, despite the fact that his research did not constitute any kind of proof of a link between the MMR vaccine and autism. Surely what fuelled the concern amongst parents was Wakefield's interpretation in the press conference before the publication of his findings, where he called for the suspension of the triple injection in favour of the single vaccines, until such time as the MMR vaccine was ruled out as a possible environmental trigger for autism and the subsequent presentation of this in the media.

The centrality of science and its experts in helping the public and policymakers make sense of the smoking, MMR vaccine and sugar risks suggests that technical experts have the capacity to influence the perception of others in both obvious and hidden ways. This view is in line with the assertion made in several studies, such as Collingridge and Reeve (1986), Jasanoff (1996) and Fischbacher-Smith (2012), that expertise is seen as a sense-making aid to other stakeholders engaged in dialogue. The centrality of science and its experts suggests that technical experts are key influential amplification agents during unfolding public health controversies, especially in the policy context. Lukes (2005) recognises that this form of power does not have to be negative but rather "productive, transformative, authoritative and compatible with dignity" (p. 109). Technical expertise has allowed us to better understand the risk we face and enabled us to build capacity by carefully and critically reflecting upon the evidence around us (Muscatelli 2016). However, where there are gaps in knowledge, and where vested interest cannot be ruled out we must pay attention to how technical experts may become prominent, and perhaps dangerous, amplification or attenuation agents.

It can be seen from the analysis of the evolving events with the three debates that the media are another source of the exercise of ideological power. For example, in the press conference before and after *The Lancet* 1998 publication of his work, and in subsequent presentations in the media, Andrew Wakefield's interpretation fuelled concerns amongst parents that the MMR vaccine may indeed be linked to autism. This assertion is in line with other studies, such as Anderson (1999), who pointed to "media scares" as being responsible for the decline in MMR vaccine uptake. Lukes (2005) has highlighted the importance of media sources and how they shape the "perception, conception and preferences" of risk in ways that may even shape public perception away from what would be in its own best interest. Indeed, expert interpretation and media sources are critical in risk communication about public health and safety since members of the public are sometimes unwilling or unable to accurately assess or decode the science or evidence for themselves.

Agency Structure in Risk Debate

Insight from Giddens' (1979) agency and structure notion of power can be seen also to be manifest in the analysis of the evolving events within the examined case studies. For example, representatives of the tobacco industry sought to shape policy developments by pursuing an informal health policy arrangement by voluntary agreement with the government on tobacco regulation. This enabled them to develop social and professional relationships with important politicians and enabled them to exchange opinions with policymakers. These negotiations, according to Collingridge and Reeve (1986), strengthened the industry political positions by enabling them to delay or make unnecessary the establishment of stricter and legally binding rules. For example, the 1971 negotiation over the health warnings on tobacco products (accepted by the government) was found to have an influence on the abandonment of a Private Member's Bill in the House of commons which threatened a much stronger warning on cigarette packs (Popham 1981).

Stakeholder relationships (between expert committees and policymakers) were also prominent within the three case study debates. For example, the 37-member expert committee stated that there was no reason for a policy change in the current MMR vaccine programme (Medicines Control Agency and Department of Health 2001), and this recommendation shaped the policy perspective taken on the MMR vaccine. As a result of this recommendation, the government decided not to take any action. This was against Wakefield's suggestion that had called for the withdrawal of the triple dose in favour of a separate single vaccine for each disease. Such a relationship can also be seen in the sugar debate to shape the recommendation to reduce sugar to 10% and 5% by the WHO and *PHE*. Such a stakeholder relationship can be seen to be frequently manifest in the sugar debate following the lead-up to the WHO recommendations and the UK-wide level of sugary products.

Resistive Power in Risk Debate

Foucault's notion of resistive power is also relevant here. This can be observed within the MMR vaccine debate in terms of some parents' refusal to give consent to their infants being given the MMR vaccine, and opting instead for the single immunisation components (Evans et al. 2001). Resistance is a power avenue of powerful influence, as can be seen by the decline in the uptake of the MMR vaccination and in the way that vaccination went below the threshold of herd immunity for the first time since the introduction of the vaccine. This exercise of power led the government to change its strategy towards communicating its position on the MMR vaccine risk. There was also a change from a one-way communication strategy focused on reassurance to a two-way and interactive communication strategy. The UK government later launched a new website, "MMR: The facts", and this enabled a two-way communication. This gave parents access to the relevant information and also enabled them to address any concerns they may have had by putting direct questions to members of the Department of Health.

The above analysis of power suggests that non-decision-making power (Bachrach and Baratz 1962), ideological power (Lukes 2005) and agency and structure (Giddens 1979), as well as Foucault's resistive power (Foucault 1978) and the power societal context influence on public debates, were together able to explain how power shaped risk communication about public health and safety as it relates to policymaking. However, none of these theories of power alone are sufficient to explain how power functions in risk communication about public health and safety. Future research in risk communication should look at consolidating insight form these forms of power to theorise and empirically validate how power functions in situations of risk and policymaking.

Economic Resource, Power and Social Amplification of Risk

It is also important how wider economic factors significantly made it possible for economically resourced stakeholder groups (e.g. tobacco companies) to act in ways that protected their interests, at least for some time, until evidence began to tilt the balance of power. Aside from forging relevant stakeholder relationships, the analysis of the evolving events in the smoking debate shows that the tobacco industry was able to use its resources (e.g. economic means) to purchase the relevant scientific expertise, and to exert influence on the perception of smoking risk while also engaging in policy development relating to tobacco cigarettes. The analysis also points to how the industry circumvented the ban on advertising in the UK through sponsorship of sporting and cultural events. It was also able to delay policy interventions with legal battles against UK government policy decisions, and by working with allies in key government positions. The knock-on effect was that despite the seeming consensus in government departments that smoking was dangerous to health as early as the mid-1950s, and pressures from advisory committees, including some members of parliament and the MRC, no immediate action was taken by the government to curb the dangers of smoking to public health. This perhaps can be linked to the tobacco industry's ability to use its economic power to its advantage in the smoking risk discussion within the public and policy domains.

Voluntary agreement was used as a means to control the regulation of tobacco products, which bought the industry time and strengthened its political positions in delaying, or making unnecessary, the establishment of stricter and legally binding rules. Most of the stricter and legally binding policy interventions were legitimised in the 1990s. Also, the industry's ability to attack the technical case made against smoking by means of technical expertise could also explain the delay in policy intervention. At least, this created doubt in the minds of the public, as there was little or no causal evidence linking smoking tobacco and lung cancer. These findings correspond with the conclusion of other studies such as Saloojee and Dagli (2000), Trochim et al. (2003), World Health (2000) and Fischbacher-Smith (2012). The relationship between economic power and policymaking has also been suggested by previous studies (Smith 1988). Smith (1988) has previously argued that "corporate bodies are able to exert considerable influence on the decision-making process due to their economic power and technical expertise" (p. 1).

Another line of argument that can be drawn from the analysis of the evolving events of the three examined case studies is that those with economic and political power (agenda control and decision-making power) demonstrated higher ability to influence the technical expertise brought to bear on risk because they often have the means or authority to acquire necessary scientific expertise in risk discussion. This can be seen in how the tobacco industry was able to engage and attack the technical case linking smoking to lung cancer via its own technical expertise. It is also evident in how policymakers through scientific committees come to make sense of a potential or actual risk. Political and economic power also enhances the ability of stakeholder groups to influence other forms of power, such as ideological and structural. For example, in 1991, the UK tobacco industry sued the UK government over the size of health warnings on cigarette packs that were made compulsory, thus using legislation and loopholes in the law to delay, restrict or influence government policies on tobacco control. In this way, tobacco companies were able to use their economic resources to buy legal expertise in the court of law to further their aim. In addition, by means of voluntary agreements, they were able to use their economic resources to strengthen their agency power position. The sugar industry in its bid to lobby the government sponsored a drinks party at the Conservative Party conference, asking policymakers to tackle obesity without any detrimental impact on the industry. These findings align with the views of Kasperson et al. (1988), who suggested that the understanding of risk is a reflection of "intuitive biases and economic interests" (p. 178).

Expertise and Social Amplification of Risk

Power can also be exercised through mediated sources (such as technical expertise or media sources) whereby the public makes sense of the risk faced, which in turn shapes its perceptions, desires and needs (Lukes 1974, 2004). In the analysis of the smoking, MMR vaccine and sugar debates, technical experts are key influential agents in making sense of the risk faced in the identification, construction and communication of the risk (Collingridge and Reeve 1986; Jasanoff 1996; Fischbacher-Smith 2012). However, a critical review of literature on 'expertise' and the analysis of the smoking, MMR vaccine and sugar debates raised some caution around how technical expertise is used as a sense-making aid in policy inquiry relating to risk. Insight from the critical review and case study analysis suggests that technical experts and the nature of interpretation brought to bear on risk signals are shaped by many factors that may allow social amplification of risk to thrive. These include the epistemology and methodological orientation of scientists (Furlong and Marsh 2010), paradigm blindness (Fischbacher-Smith 2012), intrusion (Castel et al. 2007), motivational bias (Tversky and Kahneman 1973; Slovic 1993; Shrader-Frechette 2010), organisational conditions and vested interests, as seen in the MMR vaccine debate arising from Andrew Wakefield's fraudulent claims.

The significance of these intervening variables lies in how they shape the nature of interpretation brought to bear on risk signals and how technical experts engage with other available expertise (or local expertise) in their interpretation of the risk. For example, Furlong and Marsh (2010) argued that the ontological and epistemological position of scientists shapes their approach to theory, while the methodology that scientists use impacts on how they interpret risk signals. Having said this, where there is large residual uncertainty combined with vested interests, it is possible for technical experts, who often have the privilege of authority or dominate processes of making sense of risk signals, to introduce bias into their selection and use of theories and methods in a way that may amplify or attenuate their interpretation of the risk. This also determines how and the extent to which they engage with local expertise (if they engage with it at all). Andrew Wakefield's MMR vaccine scaremongering continues to be a good example of how technical expertise and bias (brought about by vested economic interest, lies and deceit) shapes expert selection of evidence (where he cherry-picked children showing signs of autism in his study) and interpretation of risk signals. Similarly, the smoking debate gives further credence to how bias can be introduced into expert interpretation where there is vested capital interest, as observed in how the tobacco industry denied the link between smoking tobacco and lung cancer for many decades.

In an ideal modern-day risk communication, it would be expected that technical experts engage with local expertise (i.e. the expertise of those who encounter the risk in their day-to-day activities) to reduce the burden of proof on technical experts, but enhance the quality of evidence upon which decision makers and those who experience the risk can rely. This is because risk assessment decisions, as correctly suggested by Furlong and Marsh (2010) and other scholars (such as Wynne 1996; Stilgoe et al. 2006; Stilgoe 2007; Fischbacher-Smith 2012; Irwin 2014; and Welsh and Wynne 2013), are value laden. As such, technical experts alone should not to have dominance or control in risk assessment and communication decisions, especially where there is large residual uncertainty and where value at stake is high. Public debates which go beyond science help in accounting for evidence, and the nature of expert opinion when it is not over-reaching (Brown 2016). This reduces the potential for distributive inequities in risk decisions (Shrader-Frechette 2010) and the discounting of local expertise, which in some cases may prove significant in pointing to public concerns and solving gaps in knowledge (Wynne 1996; Stilgoe et al. 2006; Stilgoe 2007; Fischbacher-Smith 2012; Irwin 2014; Welsh and Wynne 2013). Therefore, we must move towards risk assessment approaches where ideas and human experiences are central in public discussion of risk (see Nováng et al. 2015).

COMMUNICATION AND TRUST AND SOCIAL AMPLIFICATION OF RISK

The influence of communication (or language) featured strongly in the analysis of the three cases in this book especially in the use of language of uncertainty. For example, in the smoking debate, representatives of tobacco companies can be seen to frequently point to gaps in knowledge, and a lack of any available causal proof. By using this language of uncertainty, the tobacco industry and likewise the sugar industry were able to attack (and attenuate) the technical cases made against smoking and sugar. According to Simmerling and Janich (2016), language of (un)certainty is "highly context sensitive" and may affect how a risk argument is received and believed. The knock-on effect as seen in the smoking debate is that it delayed the transition of the smoking risk argument towards the under-critical model, and the development of any concrete policy intervention that would otherwise have improved human health and living conditions. The importance of this has been noted by Fischbacher-Smith (2011), who highlights how uncertainty "creates problems of interpretation and speculation, but also occasionally served to heighten the uncertainty surrounding the event". In such situations, those at risk may become confused about what action to take or to avoid or from which to disengage, having been alerted to a risk issue. In other words, the public may ignore the science and associated scientific advice.

Trust and credibility were also critical in the debates under examination. For example, public health authorities such as the CHSC and SACCR were observed to have believed in the credibility of Doll and Hill's research linking smoking tobacco and lung cancer. As such, they accepted their interpretations, urging the government to raise awareness of the dangers of smoking. This was also captured in the words of Dr. Green, who, after the meeting between representatives of the tobacco companies and Richard Hill, expressed the view that "it was pretty clear to me that Mr Partridge and his colleagues felt that Hill had answered all their queries in a way which left hardly any loophole for doubt..." (ash.org.uk). (Mis)trust and credibility also featured strongly in how stakeholders responded to the arguments brought to bear on the debate around the regulation of ECs (Adekola et al. 2018). This can be linked to many years of lies, deceit and cover-ups during which the tobacco industry attempted to refute claims that smoking was linked to lung cancer and other diseases. As a result, there was a lot of suspicion around any argument seen to be of economic interest to stakeholder groups (e.g. corporate organisations) in risk discussions. The lack of trust coupled with concerns about conspiracies created tension around the risk acceptability in the EC debate, and this was a driving force shifting the vaping risk argument more towards the over-critical model (Adekola et al. 2018).

The analysis of the evolving events in the MMR vaccine debate points to the importance of trust and credibility in amplifying public and policymakers' perceptions of MMR vaccine safety. For instance, the credibility of Andrew Wakefield and his claims was called into question especially within the policy context when his evidence could not be verified by a 37-member expert committee and subsequent technical research work. His credibility was further dented when he was found to have falsified evidence to support his argument (Deer 2011), which led to his dismissal by the General Medical Council in 2010. Other factors that had implications for trust can be linked to other similar prior public health debates. An example of this is the withdrawal of two out of the three brands of vaccines used in Britain by the Department of Health due to links with mild transient meningitis (Sugiura and Yamada 1991). In addition, the anti-vaccination movement that has endured since the 1900s in Britain may have entrenched further suspicion of the MMR vaccine among concerned parents (Blume 2006).

The controversies around Tony Blair and his son Leo further highlight the importance of public trust in policymakers or those responsible for managing public health and safety. This is important from the perspective that public behavioural responses may exert influence upon the success or failure of any policy strategies adopted. The analysis of the MMR debate suggests that the reluctance of the then prime minister to reveal his son's MMR status may have contributed to steering public anxiety amongst parents who were about to immunise their infants in the face of Wakefield's suggested link of the MMR vaccine to autism.

FOUR HYPOTHETICAL SCENARIOS OF SOCIAL AMPLIFICATION OF RISK AND THE IMPLICATION FOR RISK COMMUNICATION AND PUBLIC HEALTH AND SAFETY

One key conclusion drawn from the critical review of literature and the analysis of the smoking, MMR vaccine and sugar debates is that *power may be expressed through technical expertise, control of communication and creation or destruction of trust (through scientific activities)*. Table 8.1 further highlights the importance of these factors by giving illustrative scenarios of how they shape the social amplification (or attenuation) of public health

Table 8.1 Hypothetical Scenarios of Social Amplification (or Attenuation) of Risk and Implication for Public Health

Scenario	Scientist	Media	Policymakers	Population at risk	Organisations
Over-use of power of experts by stakeholder groups with conflicting science	Not affected directly but the value of science and expertise diminishes in the eyes of (individuals, groups or policy) decision makers	Presenting conflicting information to the public, leaving the conclusions to different media outlets	Cannot use evidence well. Rely on perception and uninformed debate. Politicising policy decisions	Confused. Do not engage or disengage having been alerted to the risk issue. Ignore science (and scientific advice)	Not sure how to intervene to solve problems. Ignore the risk issue in business endeavours. Exploit the situation
Extreme exercise of salient (e.g. non-decision-making, ideological and economic and agency structural) power in risk communication	Influences the direction of science in the technical verification of risk	Some risk issues do not make it into the risk agenda, therefore leading to one-sided reporting of the risk issue	Disadvantage certain perspective in policymaking. Create scenario where policy decisions do not reflect the risk experience of locals	Science may not reflect local experience or expertise. Heighten the potential for resisting science and policy intervention	Enjoy benefits or suffer loss in the public understanding or policy perspective taken to the risk
Inappropriate exercise of power to control communication (who says what, when, how and how much)	May not understand or have the full access to evidence and interpret the risk in its totality. Increasing the potential to introduce bias and intrusions where gaps in knowledge exist	Unable to access the requisite expertise, information or evidence to make sense of the risk faced by and to the public	Cannot decode meaning in or access relevant science to make informed policy decisions	Unable to engage in risk debate. Rely on the interpretation of third-party sources, increasing chances of errors in understanding	Produce own science which may be costly to generate or rely on third-party sources to make business decisions

(*continued*)

8 THE ROLE OF POWER AND EXPERTISE IN SOCIAL AMPLIFICATION OF RISK

Table 8.1 (continued)

Scenario	Scientist	Media	Policymakers	Population at risk	Organisations
Over-use of power to create trust through science and its experts	Relied on to make sense of risk signal even where margin of error or large uncertainty exist	Re-echoing the interpretation of science as if it were the ultimate truth, creating false perception	Dangerously trusting technical experts. Reduced preparedness for emergent conditions	Dangerously trusting science and its experts in the interpretation taken to risk in decision-making	Rely on expert interpretation in business decisions
Social and health consequences	Errors in understanding the nature of risk. Undermines the value of science in risk decision-making	One-sided storytelling. Media blamed for emergent conditions and undesired behavioural responses	Delay in appropriate policy interventions. Loss of trust in government officials to protect public health	Longer period of exposure to health risk and danger due to errors in the understanding of risk	Raise moral and ethical debate (CSR) in business conduct
Positive outcome	Raises research interest and creates knowledge in certain domains of risk	Raising awareness of some potential of risk and danger	Policy consideration of (some aspect of) the risk issue	Risk awareness	Consideration of (some aspect of) the risk issue in business decisions

risk and the implication this has for public health and safety. This was done by creating hypothetical scenarios that highlight how social amplification of risk affects different stakeholder groups. This hypothetical scenario can also be used as a framework by risk regulators or experts in accessing risk within a local context.

REFERENCES

Adekola, J., Fischbacher-Smith, D., & Fischbacher-Smith, M. (2018). Light me up: Power and expertise in risk communication and policy-making in the e-cigarette health debates. *Journal of Risk Research*, 1–15.

Anderson, P. (1999). Another media scare about MMR vaccine hits Britain. *BMJ*, *318*, 1578.

Bachrach, P., & Baratz, M. S. (1962). Two faces of power. *American Political Science Review*, *56*, 947–952.

Birkland, T. A. (2017). Agenda setting in public policy. In *Handbook of public policy analysis* (pp. 89–104). Abingdon: Routledge (Taylor and Francis Group).

Blume, S. (2006). Anti-vaccination movements and their interpretations. *Social Science & Medicine*, *62*, 628–642.

Brown, T. (2016). Evidence, expertise, and facts in a "post-truth" society. https://doi.org/10.1136/bmj.i6467

Castel, A. D., Mccabe, D. P., Roediger, H. L., & Heitman, J. L. (2007). The dark side of expertise domain-specific memory errors. *Psychological Science*, *18*, 3–5.

Collingridge, D., & Reeve, C. (1986). *Science speaks to power: The role of experts in policy making*. London: Pinter.

Deer, B. (2011). How the case against the MMR vaccine was fixed. *British Medical Journal*, *342*, c5347. https://doi.org/10.1136/bmj.c5347

DoH, M. A. (2001). Combined measles, mumps and rubella vaccines: Response of the Medicines Control Agency and Department of Health to issues raised in papers published in *Adverse drug reactions and toxicological reviews*.

Evans, M., Stoddart, H., Condon, L., Freeman, E., Grizzell, M., & Mullen, R. (2001). Parents' perspectives on the MMR immunisation: A focus group study. *The British Journal of General Practice*, *51*, 904–910.

Fischbacher-Smith, D. (2011). Destructive landscapes-(re) framing elements of risk? *Risk Management*, *13*(1–2), 1–15.

Fischbacher-Smith, D. (2012). Getting pandas to breed: Paradigm blindness and the policy space for risk prevention, mitigation and management. *Risk Management*, *14*, 177–201.

Foucault, M. (1978). *The history of sexuality: Volume 1: An introduction* (AM Sheridan Smith, Trans.). New York: Pantheon.

Furlong, P., & Marsh, D. (2010). A skin not a sweater: Ontology and epistemology in political science. In V. Lowndes, D. Marsh & G. Stoker (Eds.), *Theory and methods in political science* (pp. 184–211). London: Palgrave Macmillan.

Giddens, A. (1979). Agency, structure. In *Central problems in social theory* (pp. 49–95). London: Palgrave.

Irwin, A. (2014). Risk, science and public communication. In M. Bucchi & B. Trench (Eds.), *Routledge handbook of public communication of science and technology* (2nd ed., pp. 160–172). Abingdon: Routledge.

Irwin, A. (2015). Citizen science and scientific citizenship: Same words, different meanings?. *Science Communication Today–2015*, 29–38. academia.edu

Jasanoff, S. (1996). Beyond epistemology: Relativism and engagement in the politics of science. *Social Studies of Science, 26*, 393–418.

Kasperson, R. E., Renn, O., Slovic, P., Brown, H. S., Emel, J., Goble, R., Kasperson, J. X., & Ratick, S. (1988). The social amplification of risk: A conceptual framework. *Risk Analysis, 8*, 177–187.

Lukes, S. (1974). *Power: A radical view*. London: Macmillan.

Lukes, S. (2004). *Power: A radical view*. New York: Palgrave Macmillan.

Lukes, S. (2005). *Power: A radical view*. New York: Palgrave Macmillan.

Muscatelli, A. (2016). *Post-truth an ugly word* [Online]. University of Glasgow Webpage. Available: http://www.gla.ac.uk/myglasgow/news/headline_501873_en.html. Accessed 6 March 2017.

Nováng, L., Johansson, P., & Björk, F. (2015). Challenging power in the public debate: The conversation as a commons. In *'The City as a commons' 1st Thematic IASC-Conference on Urban Commons*. Bloomington: Indiana University.

Pidgeon, N., Kasperson, R. E., & Slovic, P. (2003). *The social amplification of risk*. Cambridge: Cambridge University Press.

Popham, G. T. (1981). Government and smoking: Policy-making and pressure groups. *Policy & Politics, 9*, 331–348.

Saloojee, Y., & Dagli, E. (2000). Tobacco industry tactics for resisting public policy on health. *Bulletin of the World Health Organization, 78*, 902–910.

Shrader-Frechette, K. (2010). Analyzing public participation in risk analysis: How the wolves of environmental injustice hide in the sheep's clothing of science. *Environmental Justice, 3*, 119–123.

Simmerling, A., & Janich, N. (2016). Rhetorical functions of a 'language of uncertainty' in the mass media. *Public Understanding of Science, 25*, 961–975.

Slovic, P. (1993). Perceived risk, trust, and democracy. *Risk Analysis, 13*, 675–682.

Smith, D. (1988). *Corporate power, risk assessment and the control of major hazards: A study of Canvey Island and Ellesmere Port*. Manchester: University of Manchester.

Stilgoe, J. (2007). The (co-) production of public uncertainty: UK scientific advice on mobile phone health risks. *Public Understanding of Science, 16*, 45–61.

Stilgoe, J., Irwin, A., & Jones, K. (2006). *The received wisdom: Opening up expert advice*. London: Demos. http://discovery.ucl.ac.uk/id/eprint/1380158

Sugiura, A., & Yamada, A. (1991). Aseptic meningitis as a complication of mumps vaccination. *The Pediatric Infectious Disease Journal, 10*, 209–213.

Trochim, W. M. K., Stillman, F. A., Clark, P. I., & Schmitt, C. L. (2003). Development of a model of the tobacco industry's interference with tobacco control programmes. *Tobacco Control, 12*, 140–147.

Tversky, A., & Kahneman, D. (1973). Availability: A heuristic for judging frequency and probability. *Cognitive Psychology, 5*, 207–232.

Welsh, I., & Wynne, B. (2013). Science, scientism and imaginaries of publics in the UK: Passive objects, incipient threats. *Science as Culture, 22*, 540–566.

World Health, O. (2000). Tobacco company strategies to undermine tobacco control activities at the World Health Organization: Report of the committee of experts on tobacco industry documents.

Wynne, B. (1996). A reflexive view of the expert-lay knowledge divide. In S. Lash, B. Szerszynski & B. Wynne (Eds.), *Risk, environment and modernity: Towards a new ecology* (pp. 44–83). London: Sage.

CHAPTER 9

Best Practice Risk Communication and Conclusion

CONCLUSION

The findings from the investigation carried out in this book provide a number of perspectives on how power and expertise shapes risk communication about public health and safety. The significance of this is that powerful groups with hidden interests and agendas may be able to influence policy debates in a manner that will go unnoticed, yet may constitute a disadvantage to less powerful groups (often times, the poorer sections of society).

One way forward is more open and engaged participation of all stakeholders in the processes of risk analysis and social acceptability of risk. Policy development relating to public health and safety already relies on the use of technical expertise (Wynne 1989; Wynne 1996; Smith 1990; Irwin 1995; Fischer 1998; Funtowicz and Ravetz 2003; Stilgoe 2004; Renn 2008) as a means to make sense of the risk faced. However, using these means alone can serve to "reinforce misconceptions and misunderstandings about the nature of possible threats to public health and safe" (Adekola et al. 2017, p. 345). The empirical findings from the analysis of the smoking, MMR vaccine and sugar debates shows that there is a strong relationship between over-use of power of experts by stakeholder groups and social amplification (or attenuation) of risk. This suggests that scientific interpretations must be treated with caution and not as more reliable than they are. Moreover, there is the argument that "technical expertise is domain specific" (Schneider et al. 1989; McGraw and Pinney 1990; Smith

© The Author(s) 2020
J. Adekola, *Power and Risk in Policymaking*,
https://doi.org/10.1007/978-3-030-19314-0_9

and McCloskey 2000; Castel et al. 2007). Hence, it is importance to acknowledge a reduced validity of technical expertise where there are unknowns or large residual uncertainties or when dealing with interdisciplinary issues or wicked problems.

Since many public health risks are interdisciplinary (Fischbacher-Smith 2012), there are bound to be gaps in knowledge which may be subjected to intrusions, bias and paradigm blindness (see Chaps. 2 and 3 of this book). The significance of this (according to the analysis of the smoking, MMR vaccine and sugar debates) lies in the imbalance of power amongst the different stakeholder groups, and the ability of powerful elite groups to acquire the necessary technical expertise and other professional means to shape risk communication about public health and safety and exert influence upon public perception and policy perspectives taken to risk.

The Importance of Local (Experiential) Expertise in Risk Communication

Local expertise and those in close proximity to a risk are highly important in developing an understanding of and in framing public health problems (Wynne 1996; Stilgoe et al. 2006; Stilgoe 2007; Fischbacher-Smith 2012; Irwin 2014; Welsh and Wynne 2013), especially where there are large uncertainties or unknowns about the nature of the risk. It has been highlighted in the literature that local expertise could serve as a target for scientific research in such a way that could lead to co-production of knowledge about risk (Stilgoe 2004). It could also reduce the burden of proof on technical experts and enhance the quality of evidence upon which decision makers and those who experience the risk can effectively rely. This is important as risk assessment decisions are value laden (Wynne 1996; Stilgoe et al. 2006; Stilgoe 2007; Fischbacher-Smith 2012; Irwin 2014; Welsh and Wynne 2013). Moreover, it allows us to draw on expertise and insights that lie outside normal scientific boundaries, which could provide a unique perspective to risk that would otherwise not have been considered in a scientific setting (Stilgoe 2004).

Additionally, if the public feel a sense of disempowerment, this may discourage them from taking up public health advice. Thus, encouraging open and engaging a wider set of public participation and drawing on local expertise could ease tension around risk tolerance and acceptability debates as compromises and trade-offs associated with risk issues will be well understood by the public (Adekola et al. 2017). Local expertise, even if anecdotal, forms important steps that build or provide a viewing lens that shapes risk perception in a way that may lead to estimation of the likelihood of outcomes (Rosenbaum 2016) and bring technical data alive (Covello 2003) with careful and systematic filtering (Bates and Byrne 2007). As such, a paradigm shift is necessary from the reductionist view that considers local expertise or knowledge of those in close proximity to the risk as inconsequential or bad science, to one that acknowledges its relevance in shaping risk perception and understanding of risk (Irwin 1995; Irwin 2015). Furthermore, drawing on local expertise reinforces the view that suggests that risk assessment should consider the views of all stakeholder groups (Bennett 2010) and it is the means by which the less powerful can call authorities to account in the management of risk.

The Role of the Media

The media and academics have a role to play in ensuring a fair and balanced risk communication arena. The media play a critical role (Lichtenberg and MacLean 1991) in information exchange and sharing of expertise (Murdock et al. 2003) since the media tend to be accessible to the majority of society and are largely relied upon as a means of making sense of risk. Media sources can also have a vital influence in shaping the policy agenda as well as setting the agenda for public discussion of risk issues (Lupton 1993). Formal media outlets have a moral obligation to engage multiple levels of expertise (including the experiences and expertise of those who encounter the risk) to ensure a robust and balanced view that helps the public to make sense of health risks.

Advances in ICT and the rise of social media (Wendling et al. 2013) have further enhanced the abilities of interested stakeholders within the risk arena, by use of new ways of directly reaching the wider public and allowing more perspectives to be heard. In addition, the growing use of digital media by traditional media organisations has extended their reach (Petts et al. 2001). It is, however, more useful to think of mainstream media and social media as two parallel media sources rather than as one being more authentic than the other (Petts et al. 2001).

A Two-Way Communication

Moreover, drawing on multiple stakeholders in risk communication about public health and safety encourages a two-way communication in risk assessment and reduces the burden of erroneously trusting or relying on technical experts to make value judgements on behalf of individuals or groups in situations of risk and uncertainty. The importance of this lies in the reduced validity of expertise when dealing with cross-boundary risk issues, and this avoids the pitfall of extending margins of error for expert judgement in unfamiliar risk circumstances. Moreover, with advancements in ICT, the public is now more than ever able to seek knowledge, engage in public debates relating to science and risk, share expertise, and even challenge existing states of knowledge and assumptions. Such technological advances can reduce the extent to which information and communication can be controlled and used as means to exercise power in risk communication about public health and safety and shape policy decisions. It is also possible to use the upsurge in technological advances and social media to engage the public to identify concerns and questions, in order that these can be addressed during the technical analysis of risk. It has been suggested that where sensitive issues and public concern are addressed, the pressure for social amplification of risk is reduced (Fischbacher-Smith 2012).

The Role of Academics or Technical Experts

Academics or technical experts also have a role here. It is necessary for academics to acknowledge the relevance of local expertise (Irwin 2015) or the experiences of those who experience the risk first hand or who are in close proximity to it. This will involve recognising practices that are contrary to their own worldview. This makes science relevant to the audience it serves and presents a greater potential for communicating relevant risk messages with greater impact on the different audiences.

The Selection of Scientific Committees

It is also important to make the process of expert or scientific committee selection more transparent and open to public scrutiny. This will reduce the chances of cherry-picking experts whose opinions fit in with policy ideology and thereby bring about bias in the nature of subsequent interpretations and policy recommendations. Also, effort must be made by policy makers to avoid disadvantaging other groups by making possible stakeholder relationships that may privilege certain exchanges of views, information and ideologies in risk communication. Relevant authorities need to reach out to and build relationships with all stakeholder groups, including local experts or those in close proximity to the source of the risk, before policy decisions are made. This was seen to some extent in the vaping risk debate, where through consultation the public was able to input on decision-making relating to how ECs should be regulated (Adekola et al. 2018).

Trust Relationship

However, more needs to be done in establishing trustworthy relationships with all stakeholders at all stages of the risk (including the technical) debate. In this arena, social media plays a key role in establishing and sustaining (at low cost) relationships with relevant stakeholder groups. While social media comes with added advantages as outlined above, it must be noted that using social media (such as Facebook or Twitter) for risk communication has its own disadvantages since it can be used for political propaganda or as a way of spreading so-called fake news. When this is combined with the unwillingness of some public groups to critically investigate or research the credibility of such information, this could prove problematic in creating false public perception of risk. Therefore, risk regulators and policy makers need to make efforts to establish a social media presence, and relay reliable and credible information of what is known and not known. Social media organisations also have a role to play in minimising the use of their sites for political propaganda and spreading fake news.

Making Scientific Information More Useable to All Stakeholders

Furthermore, several steps are required to make scientific information more useable when drawing on multiple stakeholder groups, including how risk information is encoded (Bernstein 2003). Most important is the fact that the use of unfamiliar (or technical) terms may be 'intentional', designed to keep those who do not understand these codes outside of the risk debate and thereby deny them the opportunity to express their right to participate freely in political decision making (Adekola et al. 2017). Language codification has the potential to create power imbalances between actors in certain domains of risk in such a way that allows the domination of certain worldviews in policy debates relating to risk at the expense of others.

The Need to Reflect Uncertainty or Gaps in Knowledge in the Risk Messages

It is also important to reflect uncertainty or gaps in knowledge in risk messages and policy decisions. In this way it is possible to distinguish evidential knowledge from political decisions, and to understand the nature of disputes and how to resolve them. It also aids risk regulators and managers in better preparing for any emergent properties of risk.

The Need for a 'Reflective Risk Inquiry'

Finally, there is a need for a 'reflective risk inquiry'. Reflective risk inquiry allows a deconstruction of risk assessment practices – a powerful way to uncover assumptions and contradictions that guides (tacitly or explicitly) risk assessment and communication practices, moving such assumptions and contradictions from the unconscious into the conscious management psyche. Scholars such as Hilgartner (1992) have argued that risk assessment practices pay too little attention to processes by which risk objects are conceptualised and constructed. Of importance is the fact that social construction of risk does not just exist in a vacuum, but is contingent upon the social construction of risk practices that makes the construction of public health risk possible (Power 2007). A 'reflective risk inquiry' will involve questioning whether the assumptions and rationality upon which risk assessment inquiry is conducted may amplify or attenuate certain perspectives and stakeholder voices over others. This reflective approach goes beyond not only the science of risk assessment and its epistemological debates, but also the regulatory, institutional and organisational (managerial) processes in which it is embedded.

LIMITATION OF BOOK

While this book has made significant contributions to knowledge, there are some limitations that must be highlighted. First, the study uses an interpretivist philosophy and social constructionist approach. Hence, the interpretation made throughout this book is contingent upon the interpretation of the researcher and the methodology used in the analysis. In addition, the sources of data collection (published sources), which are considered one of the strengths of this book, could potentially also be a limitation. Data was collected from archival and documentary sources and was therefore not specifically produced within the context of this book. However, these sources of data were used because they contain the exact information about names, references, dates and details of events, thereby broadly covering a long span of time, and many events and contexts (Yin 2011, 2013). The use of published sources also enabled the study to capture the views and input of various stakeholders, and allowed the researcher to reflect on the debates by drawing differentially on evidence and experts. Hence, it provided greater insight on each case in such a way that available evidence was more readily comparable across cases. Despite the aforementioned possible limitations, the researcher took measures to verify the work and conclusions drawn in this book by using multiple data sources. The work was also presented at academic conferences to get feedback; moreover, the researcher has sought to address the study's limitations.

REFERENCES

Adekola, J., Fischbacher-Smith, M., Fischbacher-Smith, D., & Adekola, O. (2017). Health risks from environmental degradation in the Niger Delta, Nigeria. *Environment and Planning C: Politics and Space, 35*, 334–354.

Adekola, J., Fischbacher-Smith, D., & Fischbacher-Smith, M. (2018). Light me up: Power and expertise in risk communication and policy-making in the e-cigarette health debates. *Journal of Risk Research*, 1–15.

Bates, L. A., & Byrne, R. W. (2007). Creative or created: Using anecdotes to investigate animal cognition. *Methods, 42*, 12–21.

Bennett, P. (2010). *Risk communication and public health*. Oxford: Oxford University Press.

Bernstein, B. B. (2003). *Class, codes and control: Applied studies towards a sociology of language*. London: Psychology Press.

Castel, A. D., McCabe, D. P., Roediger, H. L., & Heitman, J. L. (2007). The dark side of expertise domain-specific memory errors. *Psychological Science, 18*, 3–5.

Covello, V. T. (2003). Best practices in public health risk and crisis communication. *Journal of Health Communication, 8*, 5–8.

Fischbacher-Smith, D. (2012). Getting pandas to breed: Paradigm blindness and the policy space for risk prevention, mitigation and management. *Risk Management, 14*(3), 177–201.

Fischer, F. (1998). Beyond empiricism: Policy inquiry in post positivist perspective. *Policy Studies Journal: Wiley Online Library, 26*, 129–146.

Funtowicz, S., & Ravetz, J. (2003). Post-normal science. International Society for Ecological Economics (Ed.), *Online Encyclopedia of Ecological Economics* at http://www.ecoeco.org/publica/encyc.htm

Hilgartner, S. (1992). The social construction of risk objects: Or, how to pry open networks of risk. *Organizations, Uncertainties, and Risk*, 39–53.
Irwin, A. (1995). *Citizen science: A study of people, expertise and sustainable development*. Psychology Press.
Irwin, A. (2014). Risk, science and public communication. In *Routledge handbook of public communication of science and technology* (p. 160).
Irwin, A. (2015). Citizen science and scientific citizenship: Same words, different meanings? *Science Communication Today*–2015, 29–38.
Lichtenberg, J., & MacLean, D. (1991). The role of the media in risk communication. In *Communicating risks to the public* (pp. 157–173). Dordrecht: Springer.
Lupton, D. (1993). Risk as moral danger: The social and political functions of risk discourse in public health. *International Journal of Health Services, 23*, 425–435.
McGraw, K. M., & Pinney, N. (1990). The effects of general and domain-specific expertise on political memory and judgment. *Social Cognition, 8*, 9.
Murdock, G., Petts, J., Horlick-Jones, T., Pidgeon, N., Kasperson, R. E., & Slovic, P. 2003. After amplification: rethinking the role of the media in risk communication. In *The social amplification of risk* (pp. 156–178).
Petts, J., Horlick-Jones, T., Murdock, G., Hargreaves, D., Mclachlan, S., & Lofstedt, R. (2001). *Social amplification of risk: The media and the public*. Sudbury: HSE Books.
Power, M. (2007). *Organised uncertainty*. Oxford: Oxford University Press.
Renn, O. (2008). *Risk governance: Coping with uncertainty in a complex world*. London: Earthscan.
Rosenbaum, L. (2016). N-of-1 policymaking—tragedy, trade-offs, and the demise of morcellation. *The New England Journal of Medicine*. https://doi.org/10.1056/NEJMms1516161
Schneider, W., Körkel, J., & Weinert, F. E. (1989). Domain-specific knowledge and memory performance: A comparison of high-and low-aptitude children. *Journal of Educational Psychology, 81*, 306.
Smith, D. (1990). *Corporate power, risk assessment and the control of major hazards: A study of Canvey Island and Ellesmere Port*. PhD dissertation, University of Manchester.
Smith, D., & McCloskey, J. (2000). History repeating itself? In *Risk management and society* (pp. 101–124). Dordrecht: Springer.
Stilgoe, J. (2004). *Experts and anecdotes: Shaping the public science of mobile phone health risks*. PhD dissertation, University College.
Stilgoe, J. (2007). The (co-) production of public uncertainty: UK scientific advice on mobile phone health risks. *Public Understanding of Science, 16*, 45–61.
Stilgoe, J., Irwin, A., Jones, K. (2006). *The received wisdom: Opening up expert advice*. London: Demos. http://discovery.ucl.ac.uk/id/eprint/1380158
Welsh, I., & Wynne, B. (2013). Science, scientism and imaginaries of publics in the UK: Passive objects, incipient threats. *Science as Culture, 22*, 540–566.

Wendling, C., Radisch, J., & Jacobzone, S. (2013). *The use of social media in risk and crisis communication*. Paris: OECD Publishing.

Wynne, B. (1989). Sheepfarming after Chernobyl: A case study in communicating scientific information. *Environment: Science and Policy for Sustainable Development, 31*, 10–39.

Wynne, B. (1996). A reflexive view of the expert-lay knowledge divide. In S. Lash, B. Szerszynski, & B. Wynne (Eds.), *Risk, Environment and Modernity: Towards a New Ecology*. London: Sage.

Yin, R. K. (2011). *Applications of case study research*. Thousand Oaks: Sage.

Yin, R. K. (2013). *Case study research: Design and methods*. Thousand Oaks: Sage publications.

The manufacturer's authorised representative in the EU is Springer Nature Customer Service Centre GmbH, Europaplatz 3, 69115 Heidelberg, Germany. If you have any concerns regarding our products, please contact ProductSafety@springernature.com

Printed and bound by CPI Group (UK) Ltd, Croydon, CR0 4YY

23/03/2026

02076402-0003